NURSE BARB'S PERSONAL GUIDE TO BREASTFEEDING

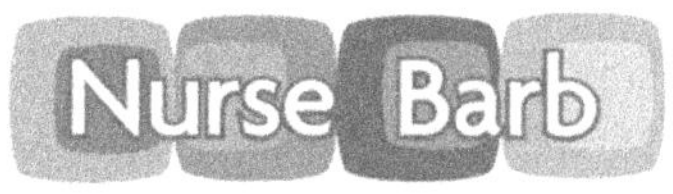

BARBARA DEHN, R.N., M.S.
Women's Health
Nurse Practitioner

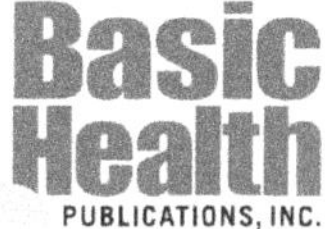

The information contained in this book is based upon the research and personal and professional experiences of the author. It is not intended as a substitute for consulting with your physician or other healthcare provider. Any attempt to diagnose and treat an illness should be done under the direction of a healthcare professional.

The publisher does not advocate the use of any particular healthcare protocol but believes the information in this book should be available to the public. The publisher and author are not responsible for any adverse effects or consequences resulting from the use of the suggestions, preparations, or procedures discussed in this book. Should the reader have any questions concerning the appropriateness of any procedures or preparation mentioned, the author and the publisher strongly suggest consulting a professional healthcare advisor.

Basic Health Publications, Inc.
www.basichealthpub.com

Library of Congress Cataloging-in-Publication Data is available through the Library of Congress.

ISBN: 978-1-59120-386-5 (Pbk.)
ISBN: 978-1-68162-758-8 (Hardcover)

Editor: Carol Rosenberg • www.carolkillmanrosenberg.com
Typesetting: Gary A. Rosenberg • www.thebookcouple.com
Cover design: Jan Davis • www.JanDavisDesign.com
Illustrations by Andrea Kelley

Contents

Introduction

Congratulations on your new baby! Whether you're eagerly anticipating a little one's arrival or have held your sweet baby in your arms, it's normal and natural to feel overwhelmed by the idea of caring for your newborn. At the top of everyone's list is the question: *How am I going to feed and care for this amazing little person and give my baby the very best start in life?* You're not alone if you're feeling like it's a lot to learn in a short time. This guide will help you navigate your way through a very special and loving journey as you learn about your unique baby and how to breastfeed.

Many moms and babies are able to breastfeed effortlessly and with very few challenges. Some babies take to breastfeeding like ducks to water; after all, they're hungry and their moms have a ready supply of milk at just the right temperature. For millions of moms, breastfeeding has been as simple as putting the baby to the breast and letting nature take its course. And yet, there are many factors that can influence every aspect of breastfeeding. Some moms have more challenges and need information, support, and assistance to breastfeed. No matter what your circumstances are, you'll need information.

This booklet is packed with answers to the most common and pressing questions every new mom has about breastfeeding: getting the baby latched on, pumping your milk, and how to solve the most common challenges, such as sore nipples, plugged ducts, what to do about leaking, and so much more.

I've also included advice about how to maintain your own healthy nutrition, tips for crying and colic, the truth about pacifiers, and important alerts for when to contact your healthcare provider or the baby's. In addition, I've provided a list of useful websites, information about how to pump and store milk, and how to find a lactation consultant in your area, as well as helpful information on baby blues and postpartum depression.

Breastfeeding your baby is a magical time that will be filled with joy and surprises. I hope that you and your baby will be healthy and happy. *Enjoy your journey!*

CHAPTER 1
Getting Ready to Breastfeed

Breastfeeding is like an intricate dance between mother and baby. Each mother's personality is unique, and every birth experience is different, which influences everything from how breastfeeding gets started in the first few days and how long a mom breastfeeds to whether she'll be able to continue if she has to go back to work. I also like to remind my patients of something that seems obvious, and many of us forget: every baby also has their own unique personality and temperament. Babies may look similar, but as every new parent knows, they quickly communicate what they like best. Within days, parents discover the way their baby prefers to be held, whether they are quiet or make a lot of noise. Perhaps your baby is active, kicking his legs and looking around, or more curious, calm, and watchful. Parents learn how their baby falls asleep, what position they prefer for feeding, and how best to get a nice burp. These are just a few of the many factors that influence breastfeeding.

There are as many variations in how babies

and mothers breastfeed as there are people! As your baby grows and changes, the way they breastfeed will also change. While everyone has the same goal—a happy, well-fed baby—there are many paths that can lead to the same destination. So trust your instincts and gather the information you need to make the best choices for your family.

THE BENEFITS OF BREASTFEEDING

Breast milk provides babies with the perfect combination of nutrients to help them grow and develop. It needs no special preparation, is readily available, and provides antibodies that help protect newborns against illnesses and infections. Moms also benefit because nursing helps the uterus contract and return to normal. Making milk requires a lot of energy and burns off extra calories, which also helps with weight loss. Sitting down to nurse a baby ensures that a new mother is getting some much needed time off her feet to rest, which helps her recover from the pregnancy and birth process.

Many factors influence your experience of breastfeeding. For some, it is easy; for others, it may be a little challenging or seem overwhelming. Most of the challenges can be overcome with practice, position changes, more rest, and patience. For other difficult challenges, working with a lactation consultant is the best way to get the expertise and help you need.

TAKE A CLASS

One of the best things you can do to prepare for your baby's arrival and for breastfeeding is to take a breastfeeding class before your due date. These classes are held in virtually every hospital and birth center around the country. To find one, ask your OB provider or midwife for a recommendation. These classes are also open to partners, which I highly recommend. When you're learning a new skill, it helps to have your family as well informed as you are. The last thing you need is well-intentioned people asking you if you're doing it right. Any mom might question her own abilities if those around her are creating doubt. So bring along your partner or any other family member who may be helping you with your new baby. It really does take a village and lots of support to care for a new baby.

In case you're worried, everyone is fully clothed during these classes and dolls are used to help new moms learn about positioning and latching on. The classes cover all the things you need to know, including how to access help should you need it after your baby arrives. Research has shown that moms who take breastfeeding classes before their babies arrive are much more likely to be able to breastfeed. Breastfeeding takes practice, and the best way to start is with a class where you can practice without the worry of a crying baby who's hungry.

BUY A NURSING BRA

Actually, buy *two* nursing bras. One to wear and one to wash. You've probably noticed that your breasts are now very different from the ones you knew and loved before you became pregnant. The size, shape, and sheer weight have changed over the last nine months to prepare for feeding your baby. In the past a DD cup might have seemed large. Now, if you get fitted, you may be in the L, M, and N ranges! Who knew those sizes even existed?

When buying a nursing bra, look for wide, comfortable straps for your shoulders that will hold up the weight of your breasts. For the back panel, the bra strap should be at least $2^1/_2$ to 3 inches wide or have at least three to four hooks for more comfortable support. Remember, your breasts will be even heavier when they're full of milk. Look for a bra that provides easy access to your breast with just one hand. If there are snaps or hooks, practice getting your breast in and out with one hand, because later on your other arm and hand will be occupied holding your baby. Because your breast size will change depending on whether you're full of milk or your baby has just eaten, make sure the cup size allows for expansion and the insertion of a nursing pad, just in case you leak milk.

You don't have to spend a lot of money to find a good nursing bra. Once you know your size, look online for good deals.

IT'S NORMAL TO FEEL OVERWHELMED

If you're worried about whether you can actually pull this off and breastfeed your baby, you're not alone. Many new mothers ask themselves the same questions: Can I do this? Will there be enough milk? Will it hurt? Will breastfeeding change my breasts? What will my partner think? It's perfectly normal to be concerned; after all, this is a new skill and involves a newborn baby who hasn't read this booklet. Most of us need practice before it becomes easier. Most women can and do produce plenty of milk, and for those who need more help, finding a lactation consultant is my best advice. Let me help by answering some of your questions.

Can You Do This?

While I can't guarantee that every mom will be able to breastfeed in every situation, I do know that the vast majority of moms can breastfeed their babies. If you go to a class, get some support and practice, chances are much better that you'll be able to breastfeed.

Will There Be Enough Milk?

Every mom worries about whether there will be enough milk to provide healthy nutrition for her baby. Most moms can and do make enough milk. I cover more about milk supply issues in Chapter 6.

Will It Hurt?

Breastfeeding shouldn't hurt if your baby is perfectly positioned and latched on correctly. You'll learn more about this in Chapters 3 and 4.

Will Breastfeeding Change My Breasts?

The answer to this question is both yes and no. Pregnancy is what causes the changes in the breasts. The hormonal stimulation is what causes the breasts to change size and shape. After a mom gives birth, her breasts may sag more than they did in the past, whether she breastfeeds or not. Women with smaller breasts may not notice much difference, while women with larger breasts may notice the effects of gravity and less perkiness.

What Will My Partner Think?

Just as every mother and baby are different, so is every partner and every relationship. Some partners welcome the changes in their relationship as everyone adjusts to a new baby. Some may need more time to transition to their new role as a parent and family. Some may feel jealous of the time and attention the baby gets from mom, and others find sharing a bit easier. When it comes to sex and intimacy, many partners are turned on by the idea of the breasts being a source of milk and others are not. The most important thing you can do is to work on healthy, respectful communication. Talk to your partner openly and honestly about what you are observing, what they might be thinking, and what you are feeling. Now that you're a family, open communication will be the best gift you can give your baby.

I DON'T WANT MY LIFE TO CHANGE

Every pregnant couple I've ever met says that they aren't going to let a new baby change their lives. They'll still be able to do everything that they used to do, because, after all, babies sleep most of the day. Before you read any further, let me just say that this booklet on breastfeeding is meant to help prepare you for the magic *and* the reality of caring for and breastfeeding your new baby. I'm not trying to scare you; I'm just trying to be the source of information that you may not have seen in other places. I'm here to help prepare you for a more realistic experience.

Believing or hoping that you'll be able to continue most of your routines is normal. Though some people might label this a fantasy, I think that any new transition in life, especially considering all that's involved with caring for a new baby, takes time to adjust to.

The reality of becoming a new parent will surprise you in ways you can't imagine. It's understandable that new parents are exhausted and barely able to get a shower let alone have the normal life they're used to. Because breastfeeding occurs six to eight times throughout the day and night, it is a full-time job! This is one of the biggest surprises for new parents. When you add up how long it takes to feed and burp a baby, and when you factor in changing a diaper, then it's almost an hour for each feeding. New babies wake up every two to three hours to eat, so by the time you've finished a feeding, settled them for a nap, gone to the bathroom, and had a glass of water, it's time to start the process all over again. No wonder new moms are tired! This is not easy and it may take a while before you begin to develop a routine for your own self-care.

One thing most new parents figure out is that now their lives are not in their control.

Not even a little bit. Where you used to be able to decide when you'd sleep, when you'd eat, and what you'd do throughout the day, as the parents of a newborn, now life rarely follows your pre-set ideas. Your babies sleep at odd hours, they seem to want to eat constantly, they pee and poop and spit up and cry, and, well, you get the idea. Often, the first sign that life is going to be different from now on is the baby's delivery, which can affect how breastfeeding gets started.

RECEIVING TOO MUCH CONFLICTING ADVICE

You're probably already familiar with receiving lots of well-intentioned and often conflicting advice from everyone about your pregnancy, the birth, and now about breastfeeding. It's frustrating to hear different opinions, tips, and advice from each person you talk to. What's even more difficult is that many experts don't agree when you ask specific questions.

With breastfeeding, I tell my patients, "One size definitely does NOT fit all!" Each mother-baby pair is unique. All babies and all moms are different. There are some aspects to feeding that are pretty simple and common with most babies, such as burp positions. Most babies will give you a nice burp when you hold them in a few simple positions; that's easy and anyone can give advice on that. And yet in other situations, such as a baby who is not gaining enough weight, there are bound to be numerous puzzling factors, such as any health issues in mom or baby, how long a baby is able to eat, whether they are latched on properly, if mom is making enough milk, and many others that will require a lot more evaluation and assistance.

You may have to try many different remedies before you find what works, and your sweet baby may surprise you by changing his behavior every few days, so that what worked in the past doesn't any longer. Flexibility is key here, and a willingness to try different approaches will help you be less frustrated. Frustration is part of your transition to parenthood. Don't worry if it takes time to figure things out. If you think of getting to the right solution as a journey, where you may have to try different routes—but you *will* ultimately get there—it can make it easier to endure the bumps along the road. We all want the same thing—a healthy, happy baby.

WHEN YOU NEED MORE HELP

If you need more assistance, then by all means talk to your midwife, OB provider, pediatrician, or pediatric nurse practitioner. Most providers have had some training and experience helping moms breastfeed. If you or they think you need more assistance, then by all means go to a breastfeeding support group at your local hospital, or contact a certified lactation consultant. Lactation consultants have the education, training, and experience to help you breastfeed your baby. They may want to watch one or more breastfeeding sessions, and then they will provide clear guidelines and techniques to help. They will also monitor and follow up on your progress. This is the best way to intervene early when the challenges are more difficult. You can call your providers for a recommendation, or go to www.ILCA.org—the International Lactation Consultant Association—to find one in your area.

FACTORING IN YOUR DELIVERY

No matter what kind of delivery you had, do take advantage of all the help and wisdom of your maternity nurses and lactation consultants in the hospital. Even if you're only there for a few days, they can show you how to hold your little one, how to get them latched on, how to troubleshoot some of the common challenges, what to watch out for, and so much more.

Practice, practice, practice in the hospital is the key to more success at home. Take advantage of the opportunities to ask questions and get assistance with any of your concerns when you have the support and knowledge of the nurses in the hospital. Many have years of experience helping moms get babies latched on correctly and breastfeeding smoothly.

Though every new mom hopes for a quick, painless delivery—where they barely notice any discomfort and a healthy, perfect, happy baby pops out easily—the reality for 99 percent of moms is quite different. If your delivery is not what you expected, then you're in good company. I wish we could all have exactly what we'd hoped for, and that our birth, our baby, and our body would do what we want, when we want. Since that's not the case for the vast majority of us, then virtually every mom you'll ever meet will have a story to tell about her delivery and how she coped with it.

If your birth experience was not what you expected, it's normal for you to need time to process what occurred and to need extra support to be able to provide breast milk for your baby. If you had an unexpected C-section, a traumatic delivery, or if your baby is in the neonatal intensive care unit (NICU), it's helpful to have the maternity nurses and lactation consultants show you how to pump, how to care for your breasts, and how to store your milk.

CHAPTER 2

The First Few Days: Your Breasts and Your Milk

When you understand how the breasts produce milk, the information and advice you receive about positioning your baby and getting a good latch make more sense. Throughout your pregnancy, your breasts were changing and adapting as they prepared for your baby's arrival. Inside the breasts, there are clusters of milk-producing cells known as *alveoli* that are connected to the nipple by the *milk ducts.* The alveoli resemble grapes, while the milk ducts look like stalks. As milk is produced, it fills up the alveoli and then travels from the alveoli down the milk ducts to small holding areas known as *milk sinuses,* just underneath the areola, which is the dark area that surrounds the nipple.

Breastfeeding is more than just putting your baby to the breast to feed. Many other things are going on at the same time that may surprise you. For one, the baby's mouth must be properly positioned over the areola to provide enough force to stimulate the let-down

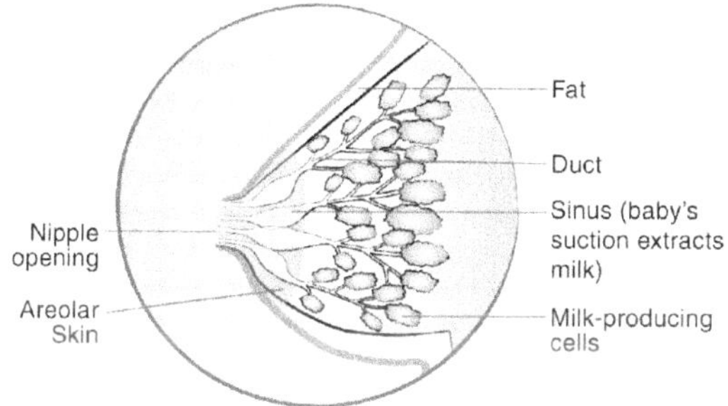

Diagram of the internal anatomy of the breast.

reflex and allow the milk to eject through the milk sinuses and the nipple. Just under the areola are nerve cells that signal the brain to produce more milk. Breastfeeding is all about *demand* and then *supply.* The baby's sucking on the areola produces milk flow immediately and also stimulates the nerves below the surface. This is part of a complex feedback pathway that, in turn, tells the brain to signal the milk-producing cells in the breast to make more milk the next day.

The pressure from the baby's sucking on the areola also sends signals to the mother's brain to release oxytocin, which is not only a "feel-good" chemical that enhances mother-and-baby bonding but also helps the uterus contract and regain its tone, shape, and pre-pregnancy size. Breast pumping does much the same thing via the action of the pump's suction over the breast and areola. For more on getting a good latch, see Chapter 4.

LIQUID GOLD: COLOSTRUM

Before your milk comes in, your breasts will produce small amounts of a thick, yellow fluid, or "first milk," known as colostrum. This is the perfect first milk for your baby and is a rich source of nourishment containing protein, fat, minerals, milk sugar (lactose), antioxidants, growth factors, antibodies, and many other nutrients. The antibodies are particularly important because they help protect your newborn from infection. Colostrum is what is produced by the breasts for approximately four to five days before the milk comes in. The amount of colostrum produced at each feeding may only be one ounce or less, which is the perfect amount for the baby's stomach; the baby's stomach is about the size of a marble and can only digest this small amount of nourishment.

It's important to put the baby to the breast frequently in the first few days. Aim to breastfeed every two and half to three hours for about ten to fifteen minutes on each side throughout the day and night. Because the baby's stomach is so small, it will fill up and empty quickly. Don't worry about the frequent feedings. As your baby grows, her stomach grows larger than a marble, and she will drink more and more at each feeding and not need to eat as often.

When you're trying to figure out when to feed the baby, keep a log of when you start and then plan to start again two and a half to three hours later. When your healthcare provider asks how often you are feeding the baby, start timing when you start a feeding and note the intervals from the beginning of one breastfeeding session to the beginning of the next.

Frequent Breastfeeding in the First Few Days Will:

- ❑ Provide ample amounts of colostrum, which acts as a natural laxative, helping the baby pass their first stools—the dark, sticky, tarry stool known as meconium.
- ❑ Provide protein, growth factors, and nutrients for your baby's growth and development.
- ❑ Provide protective antibodies that help strengthen your baby's immune system.
- ❑ Stimulate further milk production.
- ❑ Help lessen or prevent engorgement of the breasts when the milk does come in.
- ❑ Provide lots of practice for mom and baby.
- ❑ Stimulate the release of oxytocin, which will help your uterus return to normal and prevent too much bleeding.
- ❑ Promote bonding with your baby.

You may notice that your baby loses some weight while you are breastfeeding with colostrum. Most babies will lose about 10 percent of their body weight in the first few days of life, even if they are nursing frequently and getting lots of colostrum. This is perfectly normal and expected. Most babies should regain the weight by their two-week checkup.

While breastfeeding with colostrum, each day you should expect to see:

- ❑ one to three wet diapers
- ❑ one to two stools

When Your Milk Comes In

There are two types of milk released when a baby breastfeeds, *foremilk* and *hindmilk.*

- Foremilk is what the breasts release when the baby starts to nurse. This has a lower concentration of fat than what is released as nursing continues, when hindmilk is produced. The foremilk generally contains more lactose, also known as milk sugar, carbohydrates, and protein. Though every mother and baby pair is different, these are the nutrients that the breast provides to the baby in the first five to eight minutes of nursing.
- Hindmilk has a higher concentration of fat than the earlier foremilk. Babies who continue to nurse for eight, ten, or more minutes and get a nice full feeding with plenty of rich, fatty hindmilk, can go for longer intervals between feedings. This is why it's particularly important for you and your baby to breastfeed for at least eight to ten minutes and for you to try to empty your breasts. Some babies will be satisfied with nursing on just one side, others will need both sides to feel full.

While breastfeeding after your milk comes in, each day you should see:

- five to eight wet diapers
- two to five bowel movements

YOUR BODY AND BREASTFEEDING

There are many factors, especially your recovery from your pregnancy and the birth, that may affect your ability to breastfeed. While these won't prevent you from nursing, they can add more stress to the situation. One of the most common pieces of advice you'll hear is that it's important to try to relax when breastfeeding. This helps with the "let-down reflex."

However, when a mom is recovering from pregnancy and birth, relaxing might seem impossible. My best advice is to try as best and as much as you can to rest, lie down, or just put your feet up. We know that rest helps maintain milk supply; after all, our bodies can only do so much in one day, and breastfeeding requires a lot of extra energy. As you care for your new baby, it's also important to care for yourself and rely upon knowledgeable and supportive healthcare professionals, family, and friends for assistance.

Your Body and What You May Notice in the First Week:

- ❑ A sore bottom. Ouch! You may be sore from a vaginal birth and/or hemorrhoids, and it may be difficult to try to breastfeed while sitting down. Try a side-lying position, using ice packs, taking over-the-counter numbing remedies, or using prescription medications. If you're in a lot of pain, try sitting on a donut-shaped pillow or even a neck pillow to take the pressure off your bottom.

- ❏ Abdominal pain from a C-section or prolonged labor can make holding your baby and breastfeeding even with a nursing pillow too uncomfortable. Try breastfeeding while lying down and ask your partner or family to help with the baby's care until you feel better.
- ❏ Exhaustion can occur if you've had a long labor, an unplanned C-section, or from many other reasons. It's not unusual for new moms to feel too tired to breastfeed around the clock in the first few days. This is the time to rest whenever your baby is resting and to ask others to help care for the baby so that you can rest between feedings.
- ❏ Many moms also feel sleepy as soon as they begin to breastfeed. That's because the hormone oxytocin that the mom's brain releases when the baby starts to suck also leads to a feeling of relaxation and sleepiness. It's almost as if your body is encouraging you to sit down and rest while you feed your baby and to nap when they nap. Gradually, over several weeks, many moms become more used to the oxytocin release with breastfeeding and are better able to stay awake.
- ❏ If you have flat or inverted nipples, it may be difficult or impossible for your baby to latch on and to suck in the way that helps them get colostrum while also stimulating your milk production. This is a situation where pumping can help draw out the nipples and stimulate further milk supply. Many lactation consultants will recommend that moms with

flat or inverted nipples use a flexible nipple shield over the areola and nipple so that the baby has something to grasp onto.

- ❑ When moms breastfeed or use a pump, the stimulation to the areola around the nipple will stimulate the release of the hormone oxytocin, which leads to uterine contractions and pelvic cramping. This also helps decrease the amount of bleeding that occurs after delivery. The contractions help the uterus recover and return to its pre-pregnancy size. If the cramping is uncomfortable, or if you've had a C-section, talk to your provider about using an over-the-counter pain reliever. Remember this cramping is helping your body recover, so even though it hurts, it's a good thing.

- ❑ Within a few days of the baby's birth, frequent nursing leads to milk production. As the amount of colostrum decreases and your milk "comes in," the breasts may become engorged with milk. They may swell one or two cup sizes and may become so full of milk that the skin stretches, leading to hard, swollen breasts that are difficult for the baby to latch on to. The best way to prevent this is to put the baby to the breast frequently to relieve the fullness. You can pump or try to manually express some milk, or try ice packs for the pain.

  Another remedy that may seem crazy, but really works, is to place cabbage leaves inside your nursing bra. Though we don't understand how this works, it does seem to decrease the swelling and allow for the baby to latch on.

- ❏ As the milk comes in, many women describe the sensation of the milk ducts filling up and the let-down reflex as a tingling or burning sensation. Though some women don't feel anything, others may experience the let-down reflex only in the first few days, just occasionally, or each time they nurse.

Breastfeeding is a full-time job. It can take eight to ten hours each day! So in addition to all of the advice you're getting here, remember to find a comfortable place to sit or lie down while feeding your baby, rest as much as possible in between, and let go of the impulse to try and do everything else you're used to doing. The laundry, e-mails, and posting photos can wait.

CHAPTER 3

Perfect Positioning for Breastfeeding

Are you ready to start breastfeeding? Okay, first things first: I want you to be as comfortable as possible whenever you breastfeed your baby. This not only helps you relax and allows your let-down reflex to release the milk, but it also helps your baby feel more secure. If moms are calm and relaxed, then their babies will sense that and also relax. It's been my experience that babies can sense any tension or fear from the person who's holding them and then get a little fidgety and squirmy themselves, which ends up making it more difficult for both mom and baby to get latched on and the flow of milk to start.

It's very difficult to feel relaxed and calm while trying to concentrate on getting the baby latched on when they are crying and hungry, so in the first few days, watch for cues that they are getting ready to eat and then offer them a feeding. Soon you'll be able to anticipate when your baby is hungry and can get them latched on and feeding before they are crying intensely.

Try to find a comfortable spot that provides support for your back and arms. Babies get heavy, so do use pillows, an armchair, a nursing pillow, or whatever support you have available. Bring the baby up to your breast, don't lean over toward her as this will cause neck and back strain. The illustrations below will help show you where to position the baby's head and mouth for maximum comfort. Here are some of the easiest positions to try.

CRADLE HOLD

In the cradle hold, mom sits up holding the baby across her body in her arms. Together, mom and baby should make a "T" shape. The baby's tummy should be resting against mom's tummy and there should be a straight line from the baby's ear to her leg. Mom should only be able to see one side of the baby's face. If she can see both sides of the baby's face, her nipple will end up rubbing on the roof of the baby's mouth, which is also known as the palate.

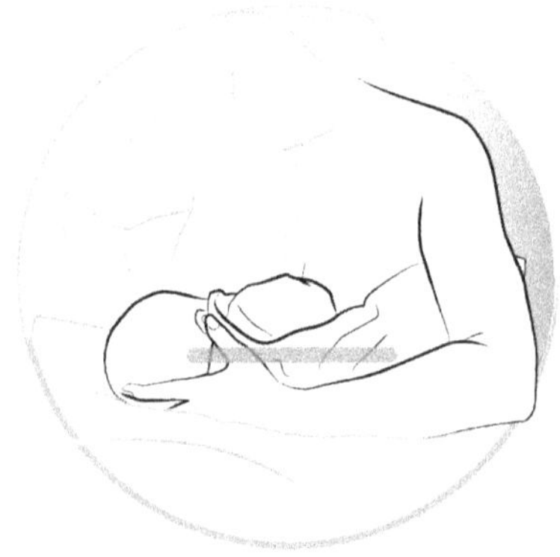

Cradle Hold

Your hand positions for the cradle hold will depend upon which breast you're offering. When offering the right breast, use your right hand to hold the breast and your left to position your baby. Once you get a good latch, you can relax your right hand's hold on the right breast and use it to stroke her head or hold a glass of water.

When offering the left breast in the cradle hold, use your left hand to hold your breast and your right hand to position your baby. Once you get a good latch, you can relax your left hand's hold on the left breast and use it to stroke the baby's head or hold a glass of water.

FOOTBALL HOLD

In this position, a mom sits up with the baby wrapped around her side toward her back. The baby's weight is supported by pillows or the arm of a chair. In this hold, the baby can either be in a straight line as pictured, or slightly angled looking up at mom.

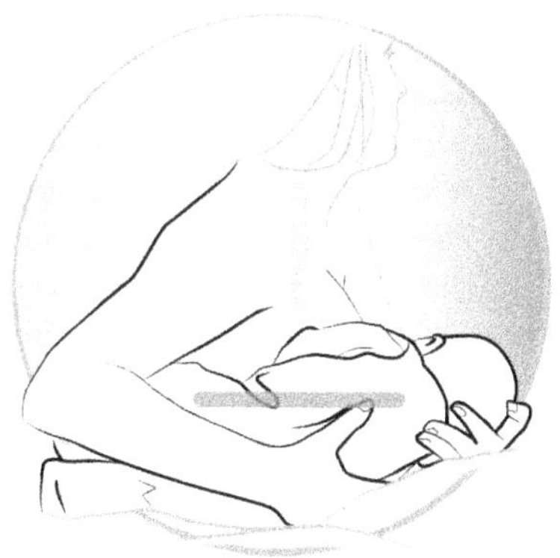

Football Hold

Your hand positions for the football hold will depend upon which breast you're offering. When offering the right breast, use your left hand to hold the breast and your right hand and forearm to hold and position the baby. When offering the left breast, use your right hand to hold the breast and your left hand and forearm to hold and position the baby. Once you get a good latch, you can relax your hold on the breast and use your free hand to get a glass of water.

SIDE-LYING HOLD

In this position, mom lies down on her side with the baby facing her. Pillows or rolled-up blankets can be used to support both mom and baby as they each lie on their sides. Mom and baby should be parallel in this position. The side-lying hold is a great way to get some rest.

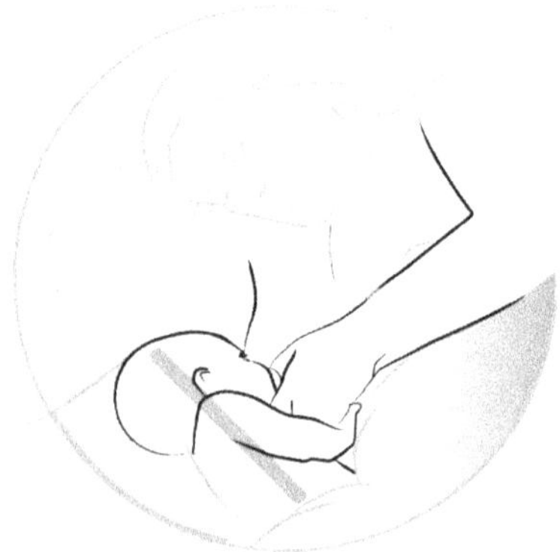

Side-Lying Hold

Your hand positions will depend upon which side you're lying on. When offering the right breast, use your left hand to hold the breast and your right arm to hold and position the baby. When offering the left breast, use your right hand to hold the breast and your left arm to hold and position the baby. Once you get a good latch, you can relax your hold on the breast and use your arm to support your head.

Breastfeeding Twins

There are many different ways to nurse twins. You may choose to breastfeed exclusively, or supplement with pumped milk or formula. Breastfeeding twins takes a lot of patience and a lot of time—it's like having two full-time jobs. Here are some tips and techniques to help:

- ❑ You may breastfeed one twin while the other one takes a bottle, and then switch at the next feeding.
- ❑ You may breastfeed them both at the same time by getting one latched on and started, and then having someone hand you the other twin to get them started.
- ❑ Moms who breastfeed twins may find that the football hold works for each twin as long as there's a lot of support on each side. Some moms use the cradle hold and have each baby's body form the sides of a V while their bottoms or their feet form the bottom tip of the V.
- ❑ There is no right way to breastfeed twins, except to do what works best for you and your babies.

❏ Often twins will be different sizes and want to eat more or less frequently.

❏ The key is to accept help whenever it's available. Taking care of just one baby can be difficult; with two it's normal to feel overwhelmed.

The more help you have, the more you can enjoy your twins and not just make it through the day. It's okay to have family and friends give you a hand. It's fun for them, too!

CHAPTER 4

Getting Started and Getting Latched

Now that you and your sweet baby are in a comfortable position, it's time to get the baby latched on correctly. The right latch will prevent pain, avoid sore nipples, help your baby get plenty of milk at each feeding, and ensure a good milk supply in the future.

WHY A GOOD LATCH IS IMPORTANT

Breastfeeding is all about *demand* from sucking, which produces a *supply* of milk—immediately and in the future. Each time you breastfeed your baby or pump your milk, there's a complex series of events happening just below the surface of the skin. Remember, the baby's mouth must cover the areola in order to force the milk out from the nipple. Their mouth should cover the areola, not the nipple, for several reasons:

1. The skin on the areola is much tougher than the delicate skin on the nipple. If a baby just sucks on the nipple, it will hurt.

2. Just below the areola the milk ducts widen

to create small milk sinuses. Small amounts of milk collect here before being ejected through the nipple. The pressure of the baby's mouth over the areola will initiate the "let-down reflex" and start the flow of milk through the milk sinuses and the nipple.

3. The pressure of the baby's mouth on the areola will also stimulate the flow of the "feel-good" hormone oxytocin, which helps moms relax and enhances bonding with the baby.

4. Oxytocin also stimulates the uterus to contract, which helps it return to its normal size and decreases postpartum bleeding.

5. Pressure on the areola will also send signals to the brain to produce the hormone *prolactin,* which stimulates more milk production in the next twenty-four to seventy-two hours.

HOW TO GET A GOOD LATCH

In order to get the baby's mouth positioned correctly, they have to open wide enough so that their mouth covers at least an inch of the areola. Just underneath the areola are the milk sinuses, or little lakes that store the milk before it is forced through the nipple. Pressure on the areola forces the milk out. Babies who latch on to just the nipple won't get a full feeding, and mom will get sore, painful nipples. Here's a two-step approach to getting a good latch.

Use a gentle tickle. You can use a finger or your nipple to lightly brush against the baby's lips or their cheek. This gentle tickle will trigger your baby to open his mouth up wide. As you watch, you may notice that the baby seems to be yawning, and because this only lasts a few seconds, it's essential to be ready to position the baby properly.

Move quickly. As soon as she opens her mouth nice and wide, quickly pull your baby to your breast so that her mouth takes in the areola and nipple. You have to be quick before she closes her mouth. Most moms need a few days of practice before this step gets easier. Your baby's chin and nose should be resting against the breast and her lips flanged out. Her nose will flare out to breathe, but if it's blocked by the breast, then readjust your position so that her nose is pulled back away from the breast enough for breathing.

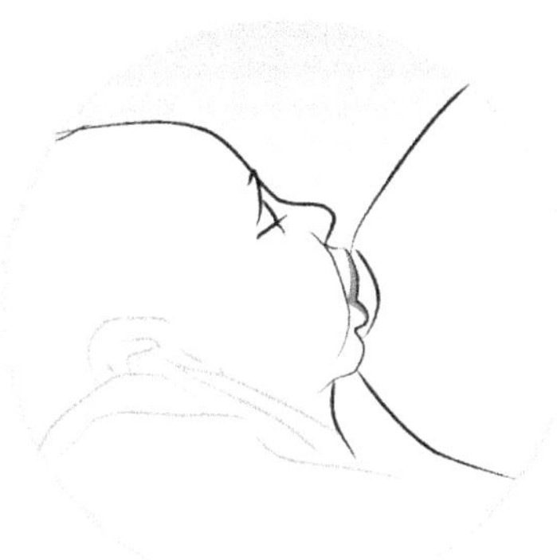

Baby at the breast with lips flanged

YOUR BABY SHOULD SUCK AND SWALLOW

The baby should take two to three sucks and then swallow. As he swallows, watch his cheeks and ears for signs of movement. If you hear a clicking noise, then he's not latched on well, and you'll need to readjust his position. Also, watch your baby for clues that his hunger is being satisfied. When there is a good flow of milk, he will be content and focused on feeding, swallowing regularly. If the baby is fussy, fidgets, shakes his head, cries or pulls away, then you may need to readjust your positioning. These are all cues that the milk isn't flowing or he's not able to coordinate his sucking. When this happens, just break the suction and start again.

YOU SHOULD HAVE NO PAIN

The nipple should point straight back into the baby's mouth. If it's rubbing on your baby's tongue or the roof of his mouth, it will be painful for you and lead to sore nipples. Pain will also occur if the baby is not positioned correctly, if they become too heavy to hold in the right position, or if they pull away from the breast. If you're experiencing pain, then break the suction and try again. It's normal

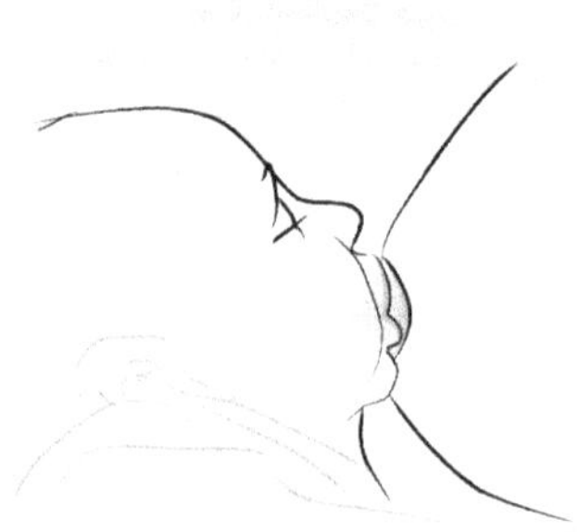

Baby breastfeeding with nipple straight back into mouth

and expected that you'll need to do this often in the first few days, but as you become more experienced this will happen less and less often. See the illustration on the previous page: this is how the baby's mouth should be positioned over the nipple, areola, and breast to ensure a painless flow of milk.

A GOOD LATCH MEANS GOOD SUCTION

To get an idea of how strong your baby sucks, try inserting a clean fingertip into her mouth. You may be amazed at the amount of pressure that your nipple and areola receive. This is why it's essential to get a good latch; the nipple's tender tissue is damaged easily, which leads to more challenges with breastfeeding.

BREAKING THE SUCTION

If your baby stops nursing on his own, his mouth will open and you can easily and safely remove the nipple. If you need to reposition the nipple during a feeding or your latch isn't just right, then you'll need to gently break the suction to avoid damaging the nipple and areola. Please don't pull your nipple out without relieving or breaking the suction, otherwise it will hurt both now and later. To break the suction, you can try any of these techniques:

- Gently insert your finger into the corner of his mouth
- Gently pull down on his chin
- Press on the part of the breast closest to his mouth

Painful Breastfeeding: Why You Shouldn't "Tough It Out"

It's critically important *not* to try to endure pain with breastfeeding. Improper positioning will lead to pain, not just with this feeding, but also with future feedings. If the nipples get raw or become so painful that even the thought of feeding the baby makes you cringe and worry about possible pain, then it will be difficult to relax enough for the let-down reflex to start the flow of milk. If the baby is sucking on the nipple or your nipple is rubbing against the roof of the baby's mouth, there's an increased chance that the delicate skin of the nipple can crack, tear, or even be rubbed off. Any small break in the skin can lead to an infection, which is known as mastitis. If you're experiencing pain, then get help with your positioning from your health-care provider or a certified lactation consultant to prevent the situation from becoming worse.

CHAPTER 5

Eating Healthy When You're Breastfeeding

They say that you are what you eat, and in this case both you and your baby will benefit from a healthy diet with lots of variety. In pregnancy, you were eating for two. Now, while breastfeeding, it's recommended that each day moms consume an extra 200 to 300 calories over what they ate while pregnant. Even with these additional calories, many moms who breastfeed and maintain a healthy diet will continue to lose between one-half to one pound each week. You should continue to take your prenatal vitamin every day, and in general you can eat any foods that you like. If your baby does seem to be sensitive to certain foods or is having tummy troubles, see Chapter 10: Colic and Crying.

HOW AND WHAT TO EAT

- Snack on healthy food throughout the day. Making milk takes a lot of energy and that means you need extra calories. You may be surprised at how hungry you are. Divide up what you're eating into five to six small meals or snacks each day. Try preparing snacks in the morning and having them available to eat later in the day to stave off hunger pangs. You could make a sandwich or quesadilla and cut it into four pieces to have ready for nibbling when you're hungry later. Or try dividing a meal up into smaller portions and saving one of the portions for a snack. Snacks may consist of a piece of fruit with peanut butter, or some cheese and crackers. Likewise, keeping small cups of yogurt, cut-up vegetables, and leftovers available makes life easier when you're busy caring for your baby.

- Drink plenty of water. Whenever you sit down to breastfeed, make sure you're also drinking lots of water. Keep water bottles filled and available so that they are available whenever you reach for one. Aim to drink six to ten glasses of water each day. Remember, you need extra fluids for several reasons. First of all, you're producing lots of fluids in the milk you provide the baby. In addition, you're recovering from pregnancy and childbirth, which involves some bleeding and loss of fluids. Many breastfeeding moms also find that they are sweating and perspiring more, especially at night. You may or may not be thirsty; however, it's important to be sure to drink plenty of fluids throughout the day and also at night if you're getting up to feed your baby.
- Power up with protein by eating at least

three servings each day. A serving is about three ounces, which is about the size of your fist. Chicken, meat, fish, eggs, nuts, lentils, soybeans, and beans are all healthy sources of protein. Your body needs protein to recover and to build more muscle mass. After all, you need strong arms to carry your baby, who is growing bigger and healthier every day from your nutritious milk. Protein is an essential building block for your baby's rapid brain growth in the first year. It's hard to believe, but soon your baby will be crawling, standing, and walking, which means he needs the best nutrition possible, not only for strong muscles and bones, but also for all aspects of his growth and development.

- Calcium is another essential nutrient that both mom and baby need. Eating and drinking three to five servings of dairy foods such as milk, yogurt, cheese, and cottage cheese each day is recommended. One cup of milk or yogurt or three ounces of cheese equals one serving. Each serving provides approximately 300 to 400 mg of calcium. Sardines, almonds, broccoli, spinach, and other green leafy vegetables also contain calcium, but in smaller amounts. When you add up what you need, it works out to 1,200 to 1,500 mg each day. Calcium is an essential nutrient for strong, healthy bones that will support your baby's ability to sit up, crawl, stand, and walk. Dairy products also contain much-needed and essential protein for your baby's strong and healthy muscles.

- If you have a lactose sensitivity or if your baby has colic, then consider getting the recommended amount of calcium from calcium-fortified juice, soy milk, almond milk, or rice milk. Many moms also need to take a calcium supplement to achieve the recommended 1,200 to 1,500 mg each day.

If You Need Calcium Supplements:

- They are best absorbed on an empty stomach.
- Don't take calcium at the same time as your prenatal vitamin.
- If you're taking any other medications or iron, take the calcium at another time.
- Do spread out when you take calcium for better absorption.
- Try taking your calcium before lunch, while preparing dinner, and before bed.

❑ Vegetables and fruits are your friends. Aim for three to five servings every day. These are essential in your diet for several reasons. They help prevent constipation, provide added fluids, and are loaded with vitamins, antioxidants, and nutrients for you and the baby. Use lots of color on the plate with salads; cooked and raw vegetables and plenty of baby carrots for snacking will also help you feel full.

Though it's tempting and seems convenient to drink five glasses of fruit juice each day, try to avoid getting your fruit from juice because of the high sugar content and the empty calories. As you try to lose your baby weight, eliminating juice from your diet will save you hundreds of calories each day. Plus, eating a piece of fruit provides pectin and fiber, which helps with digestion and helps avoid the uncomfortable and dreaded symptoms of constipation.

- ❑ Bread, rice, pasta, and cereal are all carbohydrates, which are important sources of ready energy. You'll need at least six to twelve servings of carbs each day. If you're a vegetarian, you'll need to eat fifteen or more servings of carbs each day. In either case, avoid the simple carbs like cookies, white bread, and flour tortillas, and aim to eat more complex carbs from whole wheat bread, beans, corn tortillas, cereal, brown rice, potatoes, and pasta. The trick is to make sure you're not eating too many carbs, because then it becomes much harder to lose weight and get the other nutrients you need from vegetables, fruits, protein, and calcium.

One serving of carbohydrates is small and equals:

- 1 slice of whole wheat bread
- 1/2 slice of white bread
- 1 corn tortilla
- 1/2 flour tortilla
- 1/3 cup cooked white rice
- 1/2 cup cooked brown rice
- 1/2 cup cooked beans
- 1/2 cup cooked corn, peas, or green beans
- 1 small potato or 1/2 large potato
- 1/2 cup cooked pasta

- Fats and oils are packed with energy and are important for the baby's brain and neural development. You'll need to get only four servings each day because a small amount of fats and oils goes a long way in providing energy. One serving is just one tablespoon of vegetable oil, mayonnaise, butter, or peanut butter. Because much of the food we eat already contains some fat, it's best to watch your intake.

When you're hungry and reaching for something to eat, be sure to consider how many different nutrients you're getting. A cup of yogurt with nuts and fruit stirred in gives you protein, calcium, and fruit in every bite. A turkey sandwich on whole wheat bread with cheese, lettuce, and tomato, with a glass of milk, is packed with healthy nutrients from all the food groups. Aim for lots of variety and keep drinking fluids to make healthy and nutritious milk for your baby.

CHAPTER 6

Making Plenty of Milk for Your Baby

It's normal to be concerned about making enough milk for your baby. Most moms can and do produce plenty of milk. Sometimes though, a mother isn't able to produce enough while at other times, she may be overproducing. Engorgement can occur when a mom hasn't had a chance to feed or pump, and the breasts become full, hard, and tender. This chapter covers these common challenges of milk supply and offers remedies that work to overcome them.

A DECREASED MILK SUPPLY

Within the first three to five days of your baby's life, your breasts will begin to make less colostrum and more milk. When the milk does come in, often the first thing a mom will notice is that the color of the milk is different. Instead of a yellowish color, the milk may appear more creamy and white, though it may still have a yellowish or bluish tinge.

A decreased milk supply may be apparent

from the start, with very little milk production, or it can occur if there are changes in routine, such as mom returning to work, any prolonged separation from the baby, the introduction of solid foods into the baby's diet, stress, or other causes. Anything that interferes with the frequency of breastfeeding or pumping can decrease milk supply.

Signs That Milk Supply May Be Decreased:

- ❑ The baby is fussy at the breast or cries at the breast after sucking for a few minutes.
- ❑ The baby seems to be hungry all the time.
- ❑ The baby is not producing five wet diapers and one to two stools each day.
- ❑ The baby has not gained back their birth weight by their two-week check-up.
- ❑ The baby is not gaining enough weight at their follow-up check-ups.
- ❑ Any sessions at the pump that yield less than one ounce per breast.

Babies Who Get Enough Milk Will:

- ❑ Have five to eight wet diapers and one to five stools each day.
- ❑ Gain back their birth weight by their two-week check-up.

HOW TO INCREASE YOUR MILK SUPPLY

Increasing your milk supply may be challenging, yet there are some simple remedies that can help, such as increasing your fluids, getting as much extra rest as possible, and getting help from a knowledgeable source quickly. It's also all about increasing *demand* from sucking or pumping, which should then lead to an increased *supply*. Here's a list of tips that help increase milk supply:

- Rest, rest, rest. Making milk requires lots of energy, so make time to sit or lie down while feeding your sweet baby and between feedings.
- Rest when your baby rests. Even if you don't like to nap, the more time you rest, the more energy your body can use to make milk. Avoid the urge to throw in that one extra load of laundry, clean the kitchen, or answer e-mails. You don't have to sleep, but it's important to lie down, rest, and take it easy.
- Increase your fluid intake. Aim for at least eight glasses of water or liquid each day. If you're running on empty, it's more difficult for your body to spare the extra fluid for breast milk. If you're already drinking eight glasses, try to drink an extra two or three.
- If possible, breastfeed more often. More sucking stimulates more milk production. Many lactation consultants advise putting the baby to the breast every two hours to stimulate milk production.

- Pump if possible. Use a hospital-grade electric pump. You may need to pump eight times each day for ten to fifteen minutes each time, in addition to breastfeeding or any pumping you're already doing to stimulate more production.

- Remember, making enough milk is all about *demand* first, which stimulates *supply.* Many moms will start the baby at the breast and then pump to double the amount of stimulation to the areola, thus signaling the brain there is a double demand and that more milk is needed. Think of the added demand from pumping as teaching your body to make the right amount of milk for your baby.

- Try taking fenugreek. This is a herb that's safe for both mom and baby. Fenugreek has been used for centuries to help new moms make more milk and it works. You can add it to soups, find it in teas, or take it as a supplement. We don't know exactly how fenugreek works to promote more milk production, but we do know that it's very effective. Because the amount of milk a mom makes can change overnight, I recommend that new moms keep some on hand just in case they need it.

- Recheck positioning. Be sure that your baby is positioned and latching on correctly, which ensures that the areola receives the right amount of pressure to stimulate the brain to increase milk production. If you're not sure about your positioning, then by all means ask your provider or lactation consultant for help.

- Contact a lactation consultant. When you need help, a lactation consultant is quickly going to become a trusted resource. They are credentialed, experienced, and have helped millions of moms breastfeed. A lactation consultant will ask to watch you get your baby positioned and latched on so that they can help you correct any problems and provide advice that's specific to you and your baby. To find one in your area, visit www.ILCA.org.
- Your baby needs nourishment. Talk to your pediatric healthcare provider about whether your baby needs supplementation with pumped milk or formula. They will give you guidelines for how much to offer your baby at each feeding to help them get the nutrition they need while you work on increasing your supply.

WHAT IF YOU HAVE TOO MUCH MILK?

Though many moms worry about not having enough milk, there are some moms who seem to produce gallons every day. They may be able to breastfeed and then get eight or more additional ounces from each side when they pump. Others leak throughout the day. When there's too much milk, the breasts are often engorged. If you are overwhelmed with too much milk, remember that the *supply* is influenced by the amount of *demand* and stimulation that the breast and areola receive.

To Decrease the Stimulation to Areola and Breast:

- ❏ Have the baby breastfeed on only one side.
- ❏ Pump less often and for fewer minutes.
- ❏ Use an ice pack on the breast between feedings.
- ❏ Wear a nursing bra with good support. This provides some counterpressure that can prevent the breasts from overfilling.
- ❏ When being intimate with a partner, try to limit or completely avoid any breast stimulation.
- ❏ Resist the urge to squeeze your nipples to check if there's milk present. For some women, even minimal stimulation of the breast leads to overproduction of milk.
- ❏ Try to manually express milk to relieve the pressure. Use your hands on the top or outside edges of the breasts and massage toward the nipple, while trying not to squeeze the areola or nipple area, as this can stimulate more milk production.
- ❏ Only pump to relieve pressure or engorgement and only for a short time, as any pumping will just stimulate more milk production.
- ❏ These techniques also work when you are engorged, ready to wean, or when the baby is sleeping through the night.
- ❏ Ask your healthcare provider whether you can use an over-the-counter pain reliever, such as acetaminophen (Tylenol), ibuprofen (Advil), or naproxen (Aleve), if you're in a lot of pain.

- ❑ Do ***not*** use any medications with codeine as this can build up in breast milk and be dangerous for the baby. Be sure to read medication labels and check with your healthcare provider or pharmacist if you're not certain.
- ❑ It takes two to three days for your breasts to adjust to less stimulation to decrease milk production.

ENGORGEMENT

This occurs when the milk supply increases rapidly and suddenly, which leads to the breasts becoming hard, tender, warm, and full of milk. The nipples may become flattened as the breast swells with milk. With engorgement, the baby may have difficulty latching on. The following techniques can help reduce the swelling and make the breasts less hard and more soft and pliable so that the baby has a better chance of latching on:

- Place a warm wet washcloth underneath your armpits to help with the let-down reflex.
- Gently massage the breasts with the side of your hand. Start on the outside edges of the breast and work your way toward the nipple.
- Manually express or pump some milk to relieve some of the pressure. This will help the nipple area soften enough for the baby to latch on.
- Breastfeed more frequently to prevent a buildup of milk over time.

- Apply ice packs or packages of frozen vegetables wrapped in a paper towel, pillow case, or thin kitchen towel to the breast; this will help decrease the swelling. Don't apply ice packs directly to the skin as this can freeze the skin and cause more damage.
- Wear a supportive bra that fits well. This can provide some counterpressure and prevent engorgement as well as support the added weight of the breast. Heavy, full breasts can lead to back strain and pain.
- Ask your healthcare provider whether you can use an over-the-counter pain reliever, such as acetaminophen (Tylenol), ibuprofen (Advil), or naproxen (Aleve), if you're in a lot of pain.
- Do ***not*** use any medications with codeine as this can build up in breast milk and be dangerous for the baby. Be sure to read medication labels and check with your healthcare provider or pharmacist if you're not certain.

LEAKING

Many moms leak on one side as they nurse from the opposite breast. Many leak whenever they hear a baby cry, even if it's not their own. Some will leak when they so much as think about their baby. Many moms leak during sex, showering, or with engorgement. Many moms leak without any kind of noticeable trigger. No one ever tells you about this; however, leaking is quite common and can lead to embarrassing situations if you're not prepared. Here's how you can deal with leaking:

- Use your wrist or the inside of your elbow to press firmly against the breast at the level of the areola and nipple. This counter-pressure can often stop the leaking.
- Wear a breast pad inside your nursing bra. Avoid using breast pads with a plastic lining as they can prevent the nipple from drying completely and can lead to cracks, mastitis, and yeast infections.
- Be sure to let the nipples air out frequently by keeping them uncovered whenever possible. This helps prevent yeast infections on the skin and within the ducts. Airing out also helps prevent cracks from forming when the skin is always moist.
- To air out the nipples, try leaving your nursing bra open when you're home, when resting, or even as you walk around the house. Don't get dressed immediately after a shower; stay in your robe, without a bra, to let your nipples air out.
- Many moms find that they leak so much throughout the day that showering in the morning doesn't make sense because they need to shower again at night.
- Try breastfeeding or pumping before sex if the leaking interferes with the mood. In any case, keep towels handy.
- If you don't have a breast pad, try using one half of a minipad or a thin burp cloth inserted into your bra.

- Keep a spare bra and/or tops in your diaper bag for those inevitable accidents.

RAPID LET-DOWN

This occurs when there's a large or very rapid flow of milk as soon as nursing begins and the let-down reflex overwhelms the baby. When there's too much milk flowing quickly the baby can have difficulty keeping up and can't swallow quickly enough.

The baby may pull away, cry, gag, or even make choking sounds. They may spit up or have large amounts of milk running out of the sides of their mouths. This usually improves by two months of age as babies become more efficient at nursing. Until then if you have a rapid let-down or your milk comes pouring out in large volumes or very rapidly, you can try:

- Expressing or pumping some milk before putting the baby to the breast. After the initial rapid let-down in the first few minutes the flow should slow down. You can save the pumped milk in your fridge or freezer. See page 54 for guidelines about storing your milk.

- Allow the baby time to catch her breath. If she's overwhelmed with the flow, then break the suction so she can take a break, breathe, and swallow what she has in her mouth before resuming. If you're doing this repeatedly in one feeding, try pumping or manually expressing first, then put the baby to the breast.

- Try other positions where the baby is sitting up more and his head is positioned up higher so that it's easier for him to swallow.
- Burp the baby frequently, as she may swallow and gulp a lot of air with the increased flow of milk.

Yeast Infections and Thrush

Many women have heard of or had yeast infections in their vaginas but wonder how yeast could cause an infection in the breast. Yeast are organisms that are always present in small quantities on our skin. When conditions are right, such as when there's too much moisture, or a crack in the skin, yeast can overgrow causing itching, redness, burning, and pain on the skin. A mom can have yeast on her breast and nipple, or it can enter through the nipple and infect the ducts. A yeast infection in the ducts can cause a constant burning pain deep within the breast. This pain usually occurs all the time, whether a mom is breastfeeding or not, which is different from the pain many moms experience with the let-down.

Babies may also develop a yeast infection in their mouths, which is known as thrush. A baby with thrush may have white patches inside his mouth. If the baby has thrush, he may be more irritable, have more difficulty swallowing, and may also have a diaper rash, which may also be caused by an overgrowth of yeast.

A mom's breast can develop yeast from the baby or vice versa. In either case, if you are being treated for a yeast infection of the breast, be sure to ask your pediatric care provider about treatment for the baby. Likewise, if your baby is being treated for thrush, be sure that you also get treatment and try to air out your nipples more often. It's best to have a coordinated treatment from your healthcare provider. Don't use over-the-counter remedies on your breast that are designed for yeast infections in other areas of the body.

CHAPTER 7

Caring for Your Nipples

Your nipples have some of the most delicate and tender skin on your body. Any damage to the nipples can be extremely painful and upsetting. If the nipples become too sore or raw, they may develop cracks, which can lead to mastitis and yeast infections. In the first few weeks, it's critically important to maintain proper positioning to help your nipples get accustomed to breastfeeding. In addition, try as often as possible to let your nipples air out so that they can dry out completely and recover from frequent use. As your baby gets older, your nipples will toughen and will be able to withstand more pressure from the baby's mouth.

SORE AND CRACKED NIPPLES

The nipples may become red and sore or have tiny cracks that feel like a paper cut. Some nipples will develop deep furrows that bleed with the slightest touch. If your nipples are tender or painful, it's often caused by:

- **Improper positioning.** If the nipple is not straight back in the baby's mouth, it will rub against the baby's tongue or the roof of their mouth (palate). Try repositioning the baby so that her body is straight and her mouth covers the areola. If it hurts, break the suction and try again. The illustration below and the information in Chapter 4 will help you get your baby positioned correctly.

- **A baby who latches on to just the nipple and not the areola.** This is so painful that you'll know right away if your baby is only sucking on the nipple. Babies who only take the tip of the nipple in their mouth often suck even harder (ouch!) because there's not enough stimulation on the areola to get the milk to flow. They also aren't getting a full and satisfying feeding. A baby's lips should be flanged out and cover at least one inch of the areola or more.

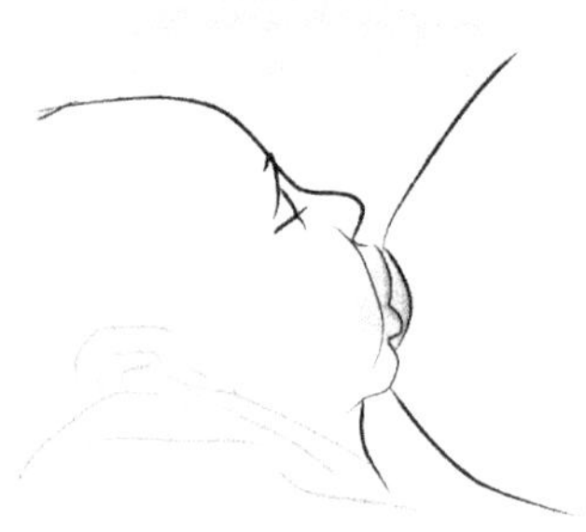

Baby breastfeeding with nipple straight back into mouth

- **A mom who becomes her baby's pacifier.** We all want to do as much for our babies as we can, and it's normal to want to try to avoid using pacifiers, and instead rely on something that's always available, like your breast. The trouble is that too much sucking can lead to nipples that are constantly in use, always wet, and never have time to air out and recover. Try to limit the time your baby sucks on each breast to no more than thirty minutes (twenty is best) at each feeding. If you want, you can offer your baby a clean finger as a pacifier. As he gets older, you can also help him find his own fist to self-soothe.

- **Pumping too long or with too much suction.** Just as constant breastfeeding will lead to sore nipples, so will any prolonged or overly frequent pumping. Give your breasts and nipples time to recover, and try to limit sessions at the pump to twenty minutes or less.
- **Too little air time for nipples.** If you can allow your nipples some time when they can get some much needed air time to dry out completely, then everyone will be happier. You can let one nipple air out while the other is engaged in feeding the baby. Or, when you have your nursing bra on for support, spend some time with your breasts uncovered. Avoid using breast pads with plastic linings. For sore and tender nipples, do try using a soothing gel or cream with lanolin.

For more information on yeast infections, see page 51. For more information on mastitis, see page 62.

FLAT OR INVERTED NIPPLES

Just as belly buttons can be "outies" or "innies," nipples can also be flat or inverted and not protrude outward. If one or both of your nipples don't protrude, your baby may not be able to grasp the areola and nipple to get milk flowing. Getting a good latch may be so difficult that both mom and baby get frustrated, leading to crying and giving up. However, it's never too late!

If you are still pregnant and suspect that you have flat or inverted nipples, and you are reading this, obtain a breast shell and wear it in your bra *before* your baby arrives. Even if you have already delivered your baby, start using a breast shell. Breast shells are two layers of hard plastic with a small hole in the middle of the side that is placed next to the breast. The hole is placed directly over the nipple. Eventually pressure on the tissue around the nipple will cause the connective tissue that's pulling the nipple inward to relax enough for the nipple to protrude outward.

Begin wearing the breast shell one to two hours each day and gradually work up to

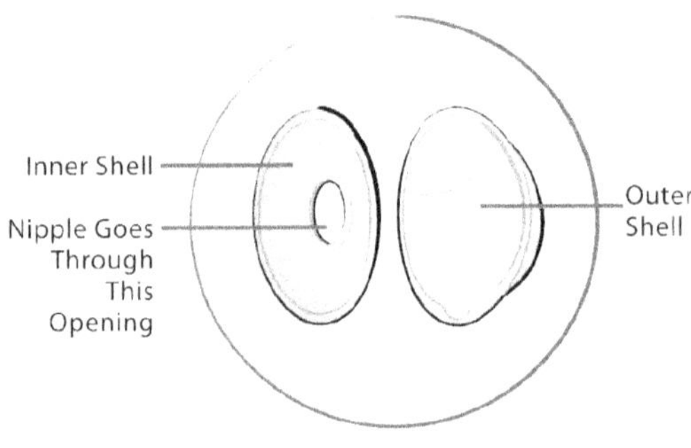

Breast Shell

using it for eight to twelve hours. If you've already delivered your baby and your nipples are inverted or flat, then wear the breast shell between feedings.

The following may also help you get your nipple to be an "outie" not an "innie":

- As soon as possible, get help from visiting with a lactation consultant.
- Pump before you offer the breast to help your nipple pull away from the breast and pop out.
- For a flat nipple, you can help the baby latch on to more of the areola by squeezing the areola just behind the nipple to help it protrude.
- For inverted nipples, place your fingers above and below the areola and pull the skin back toward you.
- Continue to offer the breast at each feeding. If the baby isn't able to latch on or suck, then be sure to pump to continue stimulating your milk supply, and provide your pumped milk through a bottle.
- Consider using a nipple shield. They are flexible, clear, silicon coverings for the areola and nipple. They are shaped like a large nipple that you'd see on a baby bottle. Sometimes nipple shields can decrease the amount of pressure that the areola receives, which can affect milk supply, which is why some experts don't recommend them. However, if using a nipple shield is the only way your baby can latch on and breastfeed, then, by all means, use it without guilt. It's

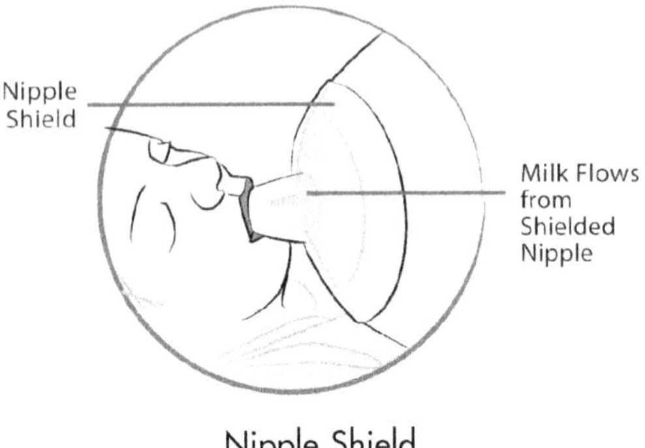

Nipple Shield

better to get the baby on the breast with a nipple shield and be able to breastfeed than it is to stop breastfeeding because your baby can't latch on.

The Brazilian Method

Here's a super secret tip from Brazil that can help if your baby can't latch on to your nipple and you can't find a nipple shield. This comes from a Brazilian lactation expert who has helped thousands of new moms breastfeed. This tip has to be secret and on the "down low" because many lactation consultants will be horrified and go into shock if you tell them that you did it and it actually worked.

If you can't find a nipple shield, grab any nipple that would normally go on a bottle and use that instead. Place it over your breast, nipple, and areola to provide something for your baby to grasp onto. Often this will help pull your nipple out and help your baby get used to sucking. Most women who have used this method only need to do it for a few days at most, until they and their baby get the hang of breastfeeding.

CHAPTER 8

What to Do for Plugged Ducts and Mastitis

By the time a baby is six to twelve weeks old, most moms and babies will have figured out the best ways to breastfeed. They are both learning from each other and most have overcome or learned how to manage the most common challenges. Most moms have developed routines while gaining confidence in all the new caretaking skills that new babies require. As babies get older and gain weight, their stomachs will grow—meaning that they will drink more at each feeding and need to eat less often. They will also start sleeping and napping for longer intervals. As babies nurse less, often a mom's breasts need time to adjust to the baby's needs. Many moms will start to notice that they are more engorged as they wait for the baby to wake from a nap or from sleeping longer at night.

HOW PLUGGED DUCTS AND MASTITIS STARTS

As we discuss plugged ducts and mastitis, it's

helpful to understand the anatomy of the breast. Inside the breasts, there are clusters of milk-producing cells known as *alveoli* that are connected to the nipple by the *milk ducts.* The alveoli resemble grapes, while the milk ducts look like long thin stalks. As milk is produced, it fills up the clusters of alveoli and then travels down through small milk ducts that join with larger milk ducts that lead to the nipple.

The small ducts are like the small streets in your neighborhood that lead to larger streets and eventually to freeways, which are much wider and where many more cars can travel.

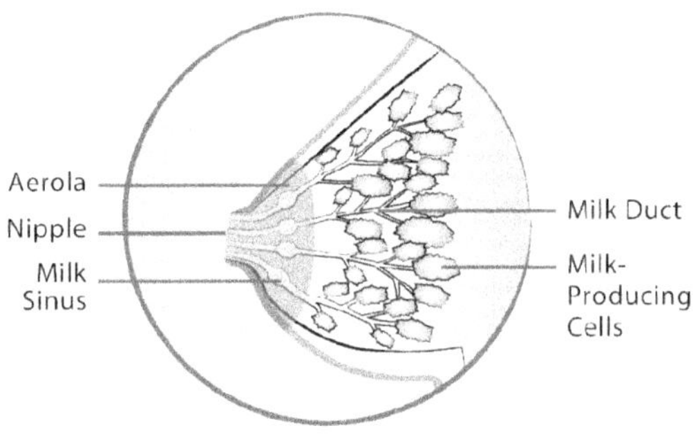

Breast tissue (side view)

When the milk stays in the breast for extended periods of time, or if there is an obstruction that clogs up the flow of milk, plugs can form within the milk ducts. Any plug will lead to an accumulation of the milk behind and above the plug as the milk that's being produced has nowhere to go. It's kind of like traffic backing up on a freeway. If the plug is not relieved, then a hard lump of accumulated milk will form within the clusters of alveoli or milk-producing cells. These will get larger as more milk is produced and has nowhere to go. Lumps from plugged ducts range in size from the size of a pea to the size of a small tangerine and may be mildly to extremely painful.

If you see white spots, bubbles, or what appears to be a tiny white blister on the top surface of the nipple where the milk ducts are located, this is an outward sign of a plug. When plugs occur at the tip of the nipple, the accumulation of milk can affect a much larger area of the breast as that larger duct carries milk from an entire section of the breast. Many moms with an obvious plug at the nipple will have pain over an entire section of the breast.

To Relieve Plugged Ducts, Try the Following:

- ❏ Continue to nurse or pump on that side. Your baby's strong suction is the best way to help get the milk flowing through the duct again.
- ❏ Place a warm compress over the lump or the area that's plugged before you start to nurse or pump to try to loosen the plug.
- ❏ As you nurse, replace the warm compress. Often the added action of the baby's sucking plus the compress will help get the plug dislodged.
- ❏ Before, during, or after breastfeeding or pumping, use firm, yet gentle massage above the level of the duct to try to increase the

pressure on the plug to help force it to move downward.

- When a plug does loosen and move down, a mom will often have a profound sense of relief within a few minutes as the pressure and pain resolve.
- Check your bra. If it's too tight or has an underwire, there may be too much pressure over a particular area, causing the obstruction, preventing the free flow of milk, and leading to a plug.
- Change your baby's position. Some moms notice that they get plugs after their babies nurse in certain positions, but not in others. This occurs because the pressure of the baby's mouth is not evenly distributed over the entire areola, which may not allow for complete emptying in some of the ducts.
- Do your best to loosen a plugged duct and get milk flowing, otherwise you can become engorged or develop mastitis—an infection in the breast.

MASTITIS

Because breast milk is a warm liquid, is full of yummy nutrients like sugar, and flows through an opening in the skin, the nipple, bacteria can easily take advantage of this situation and overgrow. If there's a crack in the skin or the milk has been accumulating from a plugged duct, then the risk of infection is much higher. Mastitis develops very quickly, is usually only on one side, and can be slightly to extremely painful.

Symptoms of Mastitis

Look in the mirror at your breasts and call your provider as soon as possible if you have any of these symptoms:

- ❑ You see an area of your breast that is more red and looks as if there's a rash present.
- ❑ Your breast is painful, swollen, and hot to the touch.
- ❑ You have a fever over 101°F or 38.3°C.
- ❑ You have an achy feeling all over.
- ❑ You feel as if you have the flu.
- ❑ You experience confusion, seem extra tired, or can't concentrate.

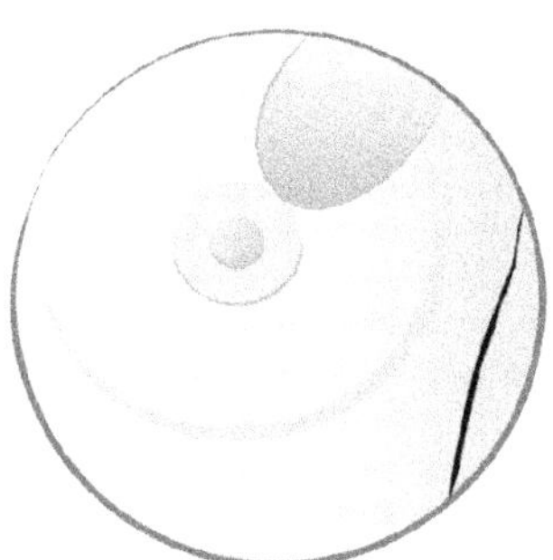

A mastitis in a wedge shape on the breast.

Treatment

It's important to treat mastitis quickly and not to wait, as this almost never gets better on its own and can interfere with your ability to continue to breastfeed. It's important to use antibiotics, as these are effective and safe for both mom and baby. Depending upon whether you have allergies, there are different antibiotics that may be prescribed. While you are being treated:

- **Continue to nurse from the affected breast.** Your breast milk will continue to produce protective antibodies, which will help protect your baby and will not cause them to develop an infection.
- **Continue to drink plenty of fluids** so that you don't become dehydrated. This will also help you continue to make plenty of milk.
- **Rest as much as possible.** Mastitis is exhausting and draining. Resting will help you regain energy and continue to make plenty of milk for your baby.
- **Use warm compresses, showers, and gentle massage.** All of these will help alleviate any plugged ducts.
- **Try changing positions.** Alternating the position and pressure of the baby's mouth may help the breast drain completely from every section.
- **Eat more yogurt or take a probiotic.** If you are taking antibiotics, then you and/or the baby may develop looser stools. Taking a probiotic or eating more yogurt can help restore the normal healthy bacteria in your system.

For information on yeast infections, see page 51.

CHAPTER 9

Sleepy Babies and Other Challenges

Some babies seem to breastfeed with ease while others need coaxing and lots of assistance. Most mother-baby pairs eventually find the techniques that work for them, yet it can take incredible patience and hard work on the mother's part. If your baby is experiencing challenges with feeding, there are many simple solutions, tips, and techniques here that may help. If you're having other difficulties or the issues are ongoing, then by all means contact your pediatric care provider for guidance and seek out a lactation consultant who can work with you and your baby and give more specific advice.

INABILITY TO BREASTFEED

Some moms and babies are unable to nurse frequently in the first few days for any one of several reasons, including a premature birth, a poor latch, sore nipples, or flat or inverted nipples. If you and your baby can't nurse during the first days, then it is essential that you use a hospital-grade electric pump to stimulate milk production and provide your pumped milk by bottle to your newborn. See Chapter 13 for guidance with pumping, and do ask your OB provider or midwife, the maternity nurses at the hospital, or a lactation consultant for help. It's understandable and normal to feel a range of emotions, from frustration and anger to sadness and disappointment, if you're not able to breastfeed your baby the way you envisioned. The tips in this chapter will help with the mechanics of providing milk if you're unable to nurse. You can also find more information on the baby blues and postpartum depression in Chapter 12.

What to Do if You're Unable to Breastfeed:

- ❑ The pump is your friend. Try to pump at least eight times each day to maximize your milk supply and keep your production up. You may feel as if you are married to the pump, and some days you will spend more time with the pump than with your baby. The reality is that if you're separated from your baby or can't breastfeed, then the pump is the only way to keep your milk production up. This takes a lot of time and energy, which means that it's important to get your rest too.
- ❑ When possible, continue to offer the baby an opportunity to breastfeed. Even if your baby isn't able to obtain a full feeding from your breast, it's often beneficial for both mom and baby to start a feeding at the breast. Many moms begin a feeding at the breast and then use a bottle of pumped milk or formula as a supplement. Others start with the bottle and finish at the breast.

- ❏ Take care of yourself. Pumping throughout the day and working on these challenges can be overwhelming emotionally. You may also feel exhausted, since you may be recovering from childbirth and caring for your newborn or other children.
- ❏ Rest, rest, and rest some more. Making milk takes a lot of energy. If you're able to nap, try to sleep whenever your baby is sleeping. Even if you can't sleep, resting helps you make more milk. Silence the phone, turn off the TV, and forget about social media, work, and the laundry. It's okay to let go of these nonessential tasks and concentrate on taking care of yourself. It's hard to care for a newborn if you're running on empty.
- ❏ You may need a nipple shield. Flexibility is key when your baby isn't able to breastfeed exclusively. Many moms with flat or inverted nipples, or those with nipple damage, are only able to get their baby latched on with a nipple shield. If this is the only way that your baby can latch on, then by all means use one for as long as you need to. See page 57 for a diagram of what a nipple shield looks like.

You may hear conflicting advice about how best to feed your baby, and sometimes it will work and sometimes it won't. Do gather information, talk to a lactation consultant, and try a variety of solutions. Get all the help that you need, and remember that it often takes a combination of techniques and tips to solve breastfeeding challenges and issues.

WHEN YOUR BABY IS SLEEPY

Each baby has his or her own individual sleep pattern. Some sleep as little as eight hours each day, and some as much as twenty-two hours each day. Sleepy babies may be hard to wake, may nurse less than eight times in twenty-four hours, and may fall asleep at the breast. A mom's breast may become engorged from incomplete emptying. These babies may also not be regaining their birth weight.

You Can Try These Tips to Wake the Baby:

❑ Unwrap and take off any *extra* blankets. Try undressing your baby and keeping them in lighter clothing and still comfortable. Don't let your baby get cold or shiver, but if it's too warm—more than 80°F degrees—many babies don't suck as well or as long.

❑ Change her diaper, make eye contact, sing and talk to her.

❑ Hold him in a sitting or upright position, being certain to support his head.

❑ Gently rub her feet, arms, back, or tummy.

❑ Gently blow on or pat his forehead with a cool, damp cloth.

❑ Wipe some milk onto her lips from your nipple or your finger.

❑ Give him gentle tummy kisses.

❑ A bath may also help her wake up.

You know your baby best and will discover what works to help him wake up without becoming too upset or fussy to eat.

FREQUENT FEEDING AND TOPPING OFF

Some babies like to nurse for five to ten minutes total for both breasts, then fall asleep and want to nurse again in less than two hours. This is also known as "topping off": when a baby's tummy doesn't empty completely, and she later adds a little bit more.

When a baby only nurses for a few minutes, she drinks mostly foremilk, the early milk that has a higher percentage of sugar, and not enough hindmilk, with lots of rich, satisfying fat. This is different from feeding a baby "on demand"—that is, when she is hungry and not on a schedule. We want to teach her to get full feedings, not partial snacks when she's hungry. When a baby wants to breastfeed frequently for short intervals, moms may experience:

- Sleep deprivation from round the clock nursing with little or no rest in between.
- Irritability, crying, and risk of depression.
- Diminished milk supply from inadequate stimulation.

If you have a full-term, healthy infant who weighs more than seven pounds, has regained his birth weight, *and* is more than two weeks old, you can use these techniques to break this cycle of frequent, short feedings that don't provide the right balance of nutrients and fat and leave everyone exhausted:

- Offer a full feeding at the breast. If the baby breastfeeds quickly and then falls asleep after five minutes, allow her to sleep.
- If your baby wants to eat again in less than three hours, then stretch the time, using distraction to wait an extra fifteen to thirty minutes, which allows his tummy to empty even more. Try changing his diaper, giving him a bath, or walking around the block to distract him and to stretch the time interval before feeding again.
- Expect crying and protesting at first, until your baby learns to take a full feeding. If the crying becomes too difficult, then let someone else hold her for fifteen minutes while you take a break and then get ready to feed her.
- While your baby may use a lot of energy protesting and crying about this new feeding routine, you're helping her get a full feeding with the right blend of foremilk and hindmilk so that she can grow stronger and healthier.
- Remember, you know what's best for your baby, and, as smart and cute as he is, his instincts to eat small amounts more frequently may not be what's best for him, and it can lead to sleep deprivation, which is not good for anyone.

ON-DEMAND OR SCHEDULED FEEDINGS

Many moms ask me whether it's best to feed their babies "on demand,"—that is, whenever they cry and are hungry—or whether it's best to put the baby on a schedule. This is a highly personal and individual preference. Some moms have the flexibility to stop whatever they're doing to feed the baby when they're hungry. This is a lot easier in the first few weeks when moms are recovering themselves. Other moms aren't able to feed their baby "on demand." They may have other children to care for, or work outside the home and need to feed the baby when they have time carved out.

Many moms wake their babies to feed them before they head to work or take other children to school. Others will offer a feeding before dinnertime so that the baby is happy and satisfied before they start meal preparation. Some moms find that after the first two to six weeks of "on demand" feedings, they can then reliably predict that their baby will be hungry every three to four hours and then can put their baby on a schedule.

There is no one right way to do this and one size doesn't fit all. My advice is to talk about your feeding preferences with your pediatric care provider so that you can determine what is best in your unique situation.

GROWTH SPURTS

When, for several days, babies nurse for longer periods of time, such as ten to twenty minutes at each breast, and/or frequently, such as every two to three hours, for several days, this is very likely to be a growth spurt. These occur on average about every three weeks. During growth spurts, babies who could last four to five hours between feedings suddenly are hungry constantly, wanting to have a full feeding every two to three hours. With growth spurts, a baby will nurse often and with more intensity to help increase your supply and his calories, as well as stimulate more milk production for the coming days and weeks.

CLUSTER FEEDINGS

Some babies eat frequently at one time of day and then have longer intervals between feedings at other times of the day, which is known as cluster or bunch feedings. With cluster feedings, babies will want to breastfeed several times within a few hours and then not be hungry for much longer intervals at other times of the day. If you feel as if you are constantly feeding your baby between 5:00 and 8:00 pm, you're not alone; many moms notice that their babies prefer to cluster feed in the evening right at dinnertime, just when they're trying to eat themselves.

Many experts believe that by the end of the day, most moms are understandably tired from a full, busy day, which can result in less time to rest and make milk. To get the same amount of calories, a baby has to eat more often. If cluster feeding in the evening is your experience, then explore these options, if possible:

- Try to rest or at least sit down in the late afternoon.
- If you're working outside the home, try to nurse your baby as soon as you see them after your time away from each other.
- Eat and drink when your baby eats.

- Have nutritious snacks such as protein bars, cut-up fruit and vegetables, string cheese, and nuts available. If you make a sandwich for lunch, make an extra and cut it up it into quarter pieces to snack on between meals.
- Hydrate with lots and lots of water.

Could It Be the Baby's Tongue?

Sucking is a natural instinct and skill that most babies started before birth. However, sucking requires coordination between the baby's mouth, tongue, and her palate. As you can see from this illustration, in order to breast-feed or suck from a bottle, the baby has to wedge the nipple between the tongue and the roof of her mouth or palate.

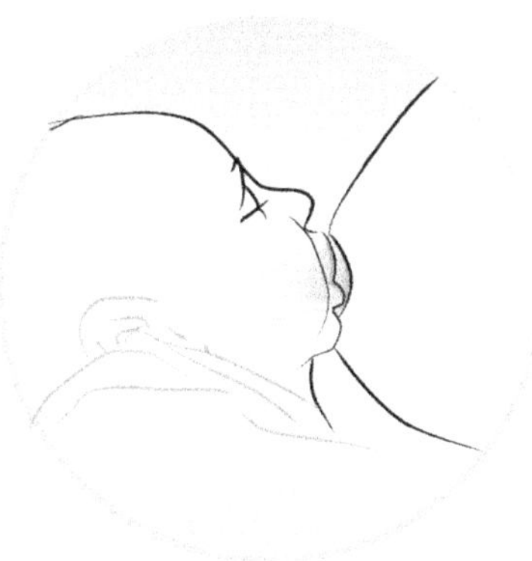

Baby breastfeeding with nipple straight back into mouth

Some babies have very long tongues and others have very short tongues. Others have learned to suck their own tongues instead of the nipple and areola. Some babies use their tongues to push the nipple away. When you factor in how nipples come in all shapes and sizes, then it's easy to see how challenging breastfeeding can be for some moms.

Babies who have been in the NICU or those who have had health challenges may have more difficulty coordinating their sucking and swallowing and often need more assistance with feedings.

If your little one seems to have difficulty, and you suspect that the baby's tongue might not be positioned properly, do get advice from a lactation consultant. In the meantime, try these techniques:

- Use the football hold. This changes the baby's direction and often keeps the tongue below the nipple.
- Gently pull down on her lower lip and chin to encourage the tongue to stay down when you get her latched
- Wait for him to open as wide as possible and then quickly bring him to the breast before the tongue can get in the way.

Tongue-Tied Babies

You may have heard of the term "tongue-tied," which refers to a baby whose tongue seems short. Some babies have difficulty extending their tongue to grasp the nipple. In these babies, their frenulum (the cord that attaches the underside of the tongue to the mouth) is tight, preventing the tongue from protruding enough to get a good latch.

Some pediatric healthcare providers or lactation consultants may recommend that you consider clipping the frenulum to help improve the tongue's mobility. This is a quick procedure that takes about a minute and can be done in a pediatrician's or dentist's office. Before you consider this, please do discuss this option with your pediatric care provider and a lactation consultant to determine if this will help your baby.

When to Call Your Provider:

- ❑ Your baby has less than five to eight wet diapers each day.
- ❑ Your baby has less than one stool each day.
- ❑ Your baby has a red rash on their bottom.
- ❑ You cannot wake the baby to nurse.
- ❑ Your baby nurses less than eight times a day.
- ❑ Your baby cries at the breast and can't latch on.
- ❑ Your baby sucks for less than five minutes.
- ❑ Your baby nurses for more than one hour.
- ❑ The mom's breasts are always engorged and the baby can't latch on.
- ❑ There is blood or pus coming out of the nipple.
- ❑ There is blood in your baby's diaper.

CHAPTER 10

Colic and Crying

Some babies will cry and be inconsolable only once in a while. Others have more tummy troubles and will cry every day for hours and hours. And despite all your best efforts and trying everything anyone suggests, nothing you do helps. These little ones may have colic. If you suspect that your baby has colic, has a lot of gas, or cries constantly, then do see your pediatric care provider as soon as possible for advice.

If your baby is gaining weight, it's reassuring, and you may have to wait a few months for his digestive system to mature and for him to outgrow his colic. Many moms find that changing their diet helps. Others switch to new formulas. In any case, do get advice from your pediatric care provider or lactation consultant. Most babies with colic feel better after three months. These can be the longest three months of your life, so do share the care of your baby with family, friends, babysitters or anyone who can give you a break from the crying. I hope that, if your baby has colic, she feels better soon; however, there are a few babies who continue to have colic for six months, so be prepared and talk to your pediatric care provider for evaluation and possible treatments.

If you suspect that your baby is reacting to something in your diet, try eliminating the suspected foods for three days to see if there is any difference. It helps to keep a food diary so that you can track any trigger foods that lead to colic. It takes about one to four hours for the food you eat to influence your breast milk.

Common Foods That May Cause Tummy Aches:

- ❑ Broccoli
- ❑ Cabbage
- ❑ Cauliflower
- ❑ Caffeine
- ❑ Chocolate
- ❑ Cows milk
- ❑ Citrus fruits and juices such as grapefruit, orange, or tangerine
- ❑ Garlic
- ❑ Nuts
- ❑ Onions
- ❑ Peppers
- ❑ Strawberries
- ❑ Tomatoes and tomato sauce

Your provider or lactation consultant may recommend other remedies such as baby's Gripe Water or simethicone drops. For babies with reflux who spit up, there may be other additional recommendations.

HOW TO COPE WITH A CRYING BABY

A baby who cries and is difficult or impossible to comfort can be your most challenging experience. As hard as this is to hear, it's important to remember that crying is her only way to communicate to you that something is wrong. You may do everything right, and your baby will continue to scream and cry. You may try the tips, techniques, and advice suggested by experts, friends, and family and have varying degrees of success. Sometimes what worked yesterday may not work today, and you may have to try new things tomorrow.

When babies cry a lot, parents shift into survival mode. They are often sleep deprived and worn-out. The important thing to remember is that *this will pass.* I promise you, your baby will not cry forever and you will get through this.

Tried and True Tips for a Crying Baby:

- ❑ **Take a few deep breaths.** If you can do your best to calm yourself first before you pick up the baby, you will feel more in control and less tense. Babies can sense tension, so the calmer you are, the more secure he will feel. Taking a few deep breaths also gives you a minute to collect your thoughts and think about how best to try to comfort your little one.
- ❑ **Swaddle your newborn.** Many new babies like the feeling of being wrapped up in a

warm blanket and tucked into someone's arms. It may remind her of how cozy it was while you were carrying her in your tummy.

- ❏ **Hold them close.** Babies feel secure when being held close to your body. They can hear your heartbeat or feel the vibration when you sing or talk to them in soothing tones.
- ❏ **Do take a break once in a while.** Often we feel as if we are the only ones who can comfort our babies and that we know best. And if you're breastfeeding, you do have the magic solution and you do know what's best for your baby. However, if your baby has been fed, their diaper has been changed, you've tried everything, and he is *still* crying and inconsolable, and, if you're feeling overwhelmed, then do take a short break. It's okay to ask your partner, family, or friends to take a turn holding and rocking the baby. Sometimes as little as ten minutes away from a crying baby will help you recharge and regain your sanity.
- ❏ **Find the motion that calms her.** Some babies respond to a slow rhythmic swaying movement, either up and down or side to side. Some babies prefer a constant hum of small rapid movements or a combination of movements. You can always spot an experienced parent because they instinctively will rock and sway with a crying baby.
- ❏ **Rockers and gliders are your friends** with a crying baby. The rocking motion has been shown in research to calm babies, and sitting in a rocker or glider will also help you stay relaxed.

- ❑ **Swings, bouncers, and car seats can save your sanity.** Your baby may like the vibration of sitting in the car, or in a vibrating bouncy seat or swing. If your baby is only happy in his swing, or he naps best while riding in the car, then do whatever you have to do to help him get the rest he needs and let go of any guilt you might be feeling.
- ❑ **Decrease the baby's stimulation.** Lower the lights, turn off the TV, and decrease loud noises. Some babies get overwhelmed by too much going on around them and have a hard time shutting it out on their own. Make it easier for them to relax without a lot of distracting sights and sounds.
- ❑ **Take a walk.** If your baby is inconsolable and you've tried everything, then try taking her for a walk in the stroller. Even if she's still crying, you'll get some fresh air, see some new sights, and her cries won't seem so loud outdoors.

WHAT ABOUT PACIFIERS?

This is a very personal choice. You may hear differing opinions from every expert, family member, or friend that you talk to. Some babies have difficulty breastfeeding if introduced to a pacifier, while most do not. A hungry baby will not be satisfied with a pacifier and will cry until you feed them. Likewise, a baby who just ate and is full may still need to suck just for fun or to help them fall or stay asleep. Experts believe that some babies need an extra two to four hours of sucking each day for pleasure or comfort, but not for food. You are the expert for your baby. Trust your instincts about whether they need a pacifier. Newborns can't coordinate their arm and hand movements enough to find their own fist to suck on until three to four months, so, until then, if they need a pacifier, you'll have to provide one or a clean finger. Here are some other things to consider as you decide what's best for your baby:

- Be a detective and look for clues from your baby. Is he a mini version of a vacuum cleaner, trying to suck on anything he can even after a full feeding?
- Is she gaining weight? If she is gaining weight and also using a pacifier for soothing, she may need more time sucking for fun. If she is not gaining weight, then it's time to talk to your pediatric care provider.
- Is he making lots of wet diapers? This means that he is getting plenty of breast milk and the pacifier is not interfering with feedings. However, if your baby isn't gaining weight and he's not making enough wet diapers, then he may not be getting the calories he needs and the pacifier may be interfering.
- Is she sleepy? Some babies who have health issues only have enough energy to suck for short periods of time and they need lots of calories to grow. These babies may need a pacifier to rest and not use a lot of energy crying, or they may not need the distraction of a pacifier. For sleepy

babies who aren't growing, do talk to your pediatric care provider.

- What happens when you don't use the pacifier? Is your baby just as happy? Can rocking, cuddling, and playing with him be just as effective to comfort and soothe him?
- Are you comfortable helping your baby learn to self-soothe? Many parents want to provide all of the love and comfort for their baby forever and ever, and yet, as they grow and develop, babies also need to learn to soothe themselves. By three to four months, most babies can find their own fist or hand to suck and self-soothe.
- What about when they're toddlers or going off to preschool? Many parents worry that using a pacifier with a newborn means that she will be become dependent on the pacifier for years and have trouble giving it up. This is a very valid concern because we've all seen it in friends and family. My advice is that babies and children change over time and what works at one stage doesn't in others. You can manage the long-term issues by being flexible, offering lots of opportunities to self-soothe without a pacifier as your child gets older, and getting help from trusted sources if you have challenges helping her give up the pacifier later.

CHAPTER 11

When Breastfeeding Isn't Going Well

Getting to know your baby and adjusting to motherhood can be a special and magical time. Most new moms are tired, they need to rest and stay cocooned with their new baby while they transition to motherhood. Rest and recovering is vitally important, but there are many factors that may make it more challenging, including a roller coaster of hormonal changes and sleep deprivation. Many moms have other children to care for or have to return to work. Others have had a difficult pregnancy or delivery or their baby may be in the NICU.

If your breastfeeding experience isn't what you wished for, if you feel overwhelmed with breastfeeding, or are ready to give up, you're not alone. Many new moms find that breastfeeding is much harder than they expected. If you are feeling any or all of these it is important to get support and help from your partner, friends, family, your OB provider or midwife, your pediatric care provider, or a lactation consultant.

You May Feel:

- ❏ Inadequate
- ❏ Depressed
- ❏ Overwhelmed
- ❏ Married to a breast pump
- ❏ Frustrated
- ❏ Like giving up
- ❏ Angry
- ❏ That your body has failed you

To-Do List

It's easy to feel overwhelmed, exhausted, and discouraged. Sometimes a little rest, help with the baby, a meal, a shower, or a few hours to yourself will give you a fresh start. Try these proven tips that have helped thousands of other moms:

- ❏ Get more rest. You'll be surprised at what a little sleep will do for you. Aim for at least six hours in a twenty-four-hour period. If you are getting less than five or six hours of sleep in a twenty-four-hour day, then you absolutely, positively need to get more sleep. Sleep deprivation leads to irritability and depression, so find ways to do less around the house, ask for some help, and do whatever you can to rest or nap. If you can get an extra one to four hours of sleep over what you're typically getting now, you'll feel so much better and have more energy to work on any breastfeeding challenges.
- ❏ Find ways to nurture yourself. If you are running on empty, you'll have less patience and become frustrated easily. Even if it's a few

minutes in a warm bath or shower, a quick walk around the block by yourself, or five extra minutes in the bathroom by yourself, it's okay to take care of yourself in order to have enough energy to care for a new baby.

- ❑ Keep to short frequent tries if you're working on breastfeeding challenges. If you spend an hour working on a particular challenge, both mom and baby will get overwhelmed. So limit yourself to no more than twenty minutes when you're trying to fix something.
- ❑ Try the simple things first. Trying a different position is often distracting enough for a baby to overcome a challenge. Make sure you're doing all the basics, like finding a comfortable position and getting plenty of rest and fluids.
- ❑ If breastfeeding is not going well and your baby needs nourishment, use pumped milk or formula supplementation as needed while you work on breastfeeding challenges.
- ❑ Find support and encouragement at a drop-in breastfeeding class or support group. Go online for support.
- ❑ Talk to a lactation consultant. You can find one at www.ILCA.org.

CHAPTER 12

Is It Baby Blues or Postpartum Depression?

Giving birth and meeting your new baby is an emotional experience. When you add lack of sleep, hormonal swings, breastfeeding, plus caring for a new baby all together, the result more often than not is the "baby blues," which is completely natural and expected.

Every mom experiences a period of adjustment and a transition to her new role. It's normal to experience some mild and minor mood changes in the first few weeks. Some new moms will notice a feeling of sadness or find that they're crying for no apparent reason. Others may have a mixture of conflicting emotions that can leave them confused and feeling guilty. They're happy to have their baby but may be confused by how sad they feel.

If the mood changes are more severe, or a mom finds that she can't sleep or care for herself or her baby, or her feelings of being overwhelmed last more than a few weeks, it may be a sign of postpartum depression. Moms who have had depression in the past, and/or PMS and mood changes with their periods, may be more vulnerable to postpartum depression. Moms who have had insomnia and sleep disturbances in the past are also at higher risk of postpartum depression. As women, our hormones do affect moods, so it's not a flaw or something to be ashamed about. More severe mood changes after a baby is born need to be evaluated so that moms can be treated and get back to caring for and enjoying their babies and their lives.

The fact is that postpartum depression is common and can be treated. The more you know, the more empowered you'll be. The good news about recognizing and treating postpartum depression is that over 99 percent of moms do recover and feel better.

Just as breastfeeding challenges can trigger postpartum depression, so can depression lead to breastfeeding challenges. When a mom is challenged by postpartum depression, it can affect every aspect of her life, especially her abilities to breastfeed and care for her baby. Moms who are depressed may not have the energy or motivation to get out of bed, to care for themselves, or to feed their little ones. They may feel so guilty or ashamed that they don't seek help or tell anyone, which can make the situation much worse.

Any time a person encounters a situation that wasn't what they had hoped for or expected, it's normal and natural to feel angry, sad, frustrated, or disappointed, which can lead to depression. If there are breastfeeding challenges on top of other issues such as a difficult pregnancy or birth, partner and family issues, a baby who might be sick or in the NICU, then moms are at much higher risk for postpartum depression. No matter what your situation, if you are concerned that you're not feeling right, do talk to your OB provider or midwife, your pediatric care provider, or lactation consultant right away.

Signs of Postpartum Depression:

- ❏ Increased irritability
- ❏ Feelings of being out of control
- ❏ Feeling sad and crying sometimes for no apparent reason
- ❏ Inability to sleep even when exhausted
- ❏ Increased anxiety and worry
- ❏ Panic attacks
- ❏ Inability to enjoy the baby or other activities
- ❏ Inability to care for yourself or the baby
- ❏ Recurring disturbing thoughts
- ❏ Obsessive behaviors, such as checking on the baby repeatedly or hand washing
- ❏ Feeling hopeless
- ❏ Feeling guilty or ashamed
- ❏ Thoughts of harming yourself or the baby

Seek help if you are experiencing one or more of the signs listed above. Contact your healthcare providers and/or a counselor or therapist right away. Here are two other good resources:

- ❏ Postpartum Support International at www.postpartum.net
- ❏ Beyond the Blues at www.beyondtheblues.com

TREATMENT

If you suspect that you or someone you know has postpartum depression, it's important not to wait for this to get better on its own. Once it is recognized, postpartum depression can be successfully evaluated and treated. Many moms with postpartum depression have an underlying thyroid condition that becomes more symptomatic after pregnancy. If this is the case and it is evaluated and treated, then symptoms get better quickly.

The good and encouraging news is that postpartum depression is treatable, and most moms will feel better with some increased sleep and also with one-on-one or group counseling. It's important to get treatment and not wait, as moms who are depressed will have a difficult time caring for their babies and themselves. Babies' personalities emerge and their brains develop from talking, cooing, and playing, which can be difficult for a mom who is depressed and only able to do the basic caregiving.

Some moms will also need medications for their recovery. The ones that are usually recommended are selective serotonin reuptake inhibitors (SSRIs) and selective norepinephrine reuptake inhibitors (SNRIs). Both are safe for breastfeeding moms and their babies. Medications help counteract the effects of hormonal changes and sleep deprivation and may only be needed for a short time. Research has shown that both moms and babies benefit, and there are fewer long-term psychological consequences when a mom is treated for postpartum depression.

Many moms who have been treated for postpartum depression say that feeling better is like opening up the curtains and letting the light shine back into their lives. They aren't just struggling to get through each day but are able to enjoy their babies and their lives again.

POSTPARTUM PSYCHOSIS

Postpartum psychosis is a rare disorder that occurs when a woman becomes delusional, has hallucinations, and loses touch with reality. It typically starts within the first week after the birth. Hospitalization and psychiatric treatment are essential since these moms are at risk for harming themselves and their babies. Moms with psychological concerns, those who are bipolar, and those on lithium before and during pregnancy are more at risk for postpartum psychosis. Call a healthcare provider ASAP if you're concerned about this for yourself or someone you know, as this does not get better with sleep or the other remedies for postpartum depression. These moms need professional evaluation and treatment. The key here is not to wait but to help these moms get the help they need immediately.

CHAPTER 13

Pumping, Bottles, and Returning to Work

The American Academy of Pediatrics recommends that moms breastfeed or provide their pumped breast milk to their babies exclusively for at least six to twelve months. Many moms are able to do this and many are not. Pumping breast milk has now become part of most new moms' experience. Many moms also find that they need to rely on infant formula to keep up with their baby's nutritional needs. Each mom's situation is unique and one size definitely does *NOT* fit all. Some moms offer one feeding of pumped milk or formula each day while breastfeeding at all the other times. Others are only able to breastfeed or use pumped breast milk once each day and use formula the rest of the time. No matter what your situation is, there's information here to help you navigate the world of pumping, bottles, and formula.

PUMPING

There are a few babies who are models of flexibility and will take a bottle anytime you offer it, no matter when or how often. If you have one of these babies, you may be able to offer a bottle of pumped milk once a week and not worry that your baby will eat. If this is your situation, you're lucky. However, if you're like many moms with a baby who prefers to stick with his routines, you may find it difficult to switch from breast to bottle unless you also develop a consistent pattern.

Most babies develop the flexibility to nurse at the breast and drink pumped breast milk or formula from a bottle if the bottle is introduced at the right time and provided at least once each day. Some babies tend to be just like Goldilocks in the story of the three bears. You can't introduce the bottle too early. And you can't introduce the bottle too late. The timing has to be *just right!*

Too early. If you introduce a bottle of pumped milk before your baby is three weeks old, it may lead to nipple confusion, with the baby seeming to wonder what this new thing is and refusing to drink from the bottle.

Too late. If you introduce a bottle of pumped milk after six weeks, your baby may be set in her routine and be unwilling to try something new. This often leads to the baby refusing to drink and lots of tears from both mom and baby.

If you know that you have to return to work and will be offering bottles while you're away from your little one, it's best to introduce the bottle prior to his six-week birthday. If you're reading this and your baby is older than six weeks, don't give up; try anyway and offer him pumped milk or formula in a bottle every day. Sometimes he'll take the pumped milk or formula better from someone other than mom, so do get help from your partner or family.

Getting Ready to Pump Tips and Techniques:

- ❑ Pump in the morning. You're likely to have more milk in the morning as a result of your rest throughout the night. Even if you were up multiple times, any rest will help you make more milk.
- ❑ To build up your supply and help your body get used to producing more milk, try to pump thirty minutes to one hour after the first morning feeding and at about the same time each day. This may not produce much milk for the first few days, so don't worry. What this does is stimulate more supply in the next three to four days.
- ❑ Regular pumping each day at the same times stimulates more supply. Remember that producing breast milk is all about *demand* first, and then *supply.*
- ❑ The percentage of fat is usually higher with early morning milk. Even a little sleep helps moms make richer milk with more fat. If you have noticed that your baby takes a longer morning nap and goes longer between feedings in the morning, it's a result of the added fat content in your morning milk.
- ❑ By the end of day, many babies nurse frequently and may be a little fussy. They may

want to eat every hour. If you're able to provide a bottle of the pumped milk, with lots of nutritious fat from the morning, around dinnertime, you may be able to alleviate some of your baby's hunger and need to eat frequently. This also gives you a little break, especially if someone else provides the bottle.

- ❏ Try to offer one bottle each day. Babies are more likely to stick with their routine and are less likely to refuse the bottle if they have a consistent experience. Some babies get out of practice if they go more than three days without a bottle.
- ❏ Encourage your partner or other family members to feed the baby with your pumped milk. Feeding a baby is a wonderful opportunity to connect and gives mom a much needed break from round-the-clock feedings.
- ❏ Many babies insist on mom, and they won't take a bottle of pumped milk if they can smell or sense that she's nearby. If this is the case, then it's a good time for you to take a shower, or take time to rest, eat, recharge, care for any other children, or get out of the house for a break.
- ❏ As you become more comfortable with pumping, you may be able to pump just before or just after breastfeeding and not need to wait thirty or more minutes. Some moms are able to pump, breastfeed, and then pump again in the morning to build up their supply.

Storing Milk

- ❏ Pumped milk may or may not separate into two layers: a thin bluish or white layer on the bottom and a thicker, yellow creamy layer on top.
- ❏ Pumped breast milk is like liquid gold. It takes a lot of time and effort to pump; so to avoid frustration from having to throw out unused milk, only store two to four ounces in each container.
- ❏ Label and date the container.
- ❏ It's safe to store pumped milk in glass or hard plastic containers, milk storage bags, or plastic bottle liners. Look for ones that do not contain BPA.
- ❏ Only keep a few days supply of milk in the fridge so that it doesn't go bad.
- ❏ Have most of your pumped milk available in the freezer to thaw if needed.

Your breast milk is safe:

- ❏ At room temp for six to ten hours.
- ❏ In the fridge for five days.
- ❏ In the freezer compartment of a refrigerator for two weeks.
- ❏ In the freezer for three months.
- ❏ In a deep freezer for six months.

When thawing milk:

- ❏ Place the container of milk in a pan of hot water that has been removed from the heat, or hold the container under cool water, gradually increasing the temperature of the water to warm.

- ❑ Shake well before feeding baby.
- ❑ Frozen milk that has been thawed can be stored safely in the fridge for up to twenty-four hours.
- ❑ Remember, babies can drink milk or formula that's at room temperature; it doesn't have to be warmed up.

Not recommended:

- ❑ Do not thaw breast milk and then refreeze it.
- ❑ Do not thaw or heat breast milk in the microwave.
- ❑ Do not place breast milk over a heat source.
- ❑ Do not place the container of breast milk in a pan that's over a direct heat source.
- ❑ Never put nipples in the microwave, as this can degrade them.

RETURNING TO WORK

Separation from your baby can be like open heart surgery without anesthetic! It's incredibly hard to be away from your baby. You may find that you're constantly thinking of your baby and can't wait to be with them again. Many moms are sleep deprived and overwhelmed by trying to work, breastfeed, pump, care for themselves, care for their babies, and try to enjoy their days, not just get through them. This is definitely a time when "good" is "good enough." Whether you're working full- or part-time, in the home or in another setting, have help at home or are doing everything yourself, most moms are exhausted from having way too much to do, so please find ways to prioritize yourself and your baby and let other nonessential things go. There's plenty of time to clean the house when your child grows up and goes to school, so please don't sweat the small stuff now.

PUMPING AT WORK

If you'll be away from the baby for more than four hours at a time, and you want to continue to provide breast milk to your baby, you'll need to pump your milk at least once each day. You may have to find time and take breaks from work to pump two or three times each day. Pumping frequently throughout the day will help you make more milk and will also help prevent engorgement and leaking.

Here are some tips if you have to return to work.

- Begin a pumping routine at least two weeks before you return to work.
- Every three to four days, substitute one bottle feeding, either pumped milk or formula, for a session at the breast. Time these substitutions for feedings that would occur during work hours.
- Don't stop all the breastfeeding at once or you will be engorged and in a lot of pain. Give yourself and your breasts plenty of time to adjust to the work schedule.

- Try to nurse and also pump before you go to work.
- Nurse as soon as you return home. This is a lovely way to reconnect and rest.
- On weekends and days off, stay on your work schedule of feedings and pumping as much as possible.
- Be sure to get plenty of fluids and rest to help keep your milk supply up.

RETURNING TO WORK WITHOUT PUMPING

For many women who return to work, the opportunity or desire to pump is not an option. If you work in a place that doesn't provide regular breaks or a place where you can pump in private, your options are more limited. Many employers do have policies in place that provide for breastfeeding moms, allowing them the time they need to pump. Do talk to your human resources person, read your employee manual to understand your rights, and work with your employer to find some flexibility.

Many moms who drive to work can use a portable pump that plugs into the adaptor in the car. As tempting as it is to multitask, please don't try to pump while driving; instead, think of your car as your private office, where you can park in the location of your choice and pump discreetly. For women who use public transportation and don't have access to a private spot at work, finding a clean restroom with an electric outlet for their pump can be too much of a challenge. For other moms, there isn't a practical solution and they decide to breastfeed or pump at home only.

For moms who can't pump when they're away from their baby, they still can continue to nurse their babies at the times when they'll be together. This is known as "minimal breastfeeding" and means that the babies have formula when their moms are at work and then breastfeed when mom and baby can be together. On weekends and days off, a mom should stay on her workday schedule. By keeping to her schedule, the breasts are "trained" to make milk at certain times during the day.

If you know that you won't be able to pump when you return to work, try to pump and freeze as much milk as you can before your return to your job. Get your baby used to the taste of formula before your first day back to work, and then do your best. The most important thing for every mom is to do the best they can, be realistic, and *not* feel guilty.

Any breastfeeding is good breastfeeding. So even if it's only once each day, then enjoy that time with your little one, knowing that the infant formulas available now are providing your baby with healthy nutrition so that they can grow.

PREPARING FORMULA

- Before you prepare formula, have all the supplies and ingredients ready—the bottles, nipples, water, and formula.
- Use clean, washed bottles and nipples.

- Read the labels and check the expiration date on the formula powder or liquid.
- Wash your hands.
- Only use the measuring scoop, cup, or device that's provided with the formula.
- Measure the formula and water exactly as directed on the packaging.
- Mix and store the formula as directed on the packaging.
- Never heat formula or breast milk in the microwave, as the heat can be uneven and too hot for the baby.
- Remember babies can drink milk or formula that's at room temperature.
- Never put nipples in the microwave, as this can degrade them.

Caution: Homemade Formula

Though some websites offer homemade infant formula recipes as a breast-milk substitute, using these instead of infant formulas that are commercially available is very dangerous for your baby's overall growth and development, and you should never try to make your own formula at home. It's impossible to replicate your breast milk from pantry items. Your baby's brain is doubling in size in the first year, which means that he needs a precise blend of nutrients, fat, protein, calcium, and vitamins. There's no way you or anyone online can possibly mix up the proper amounts of carbohydrates and the right blend of fats, vitamins, and nutrients that your baby's stomach can absorb in the correct ratios from items in your kitchen or grocery store. Commercially available infant formula is the only safe substitute for breast milk. Don't be tempted to make your own formula, as this can have very dangerous and long-lasting, permanent consequences for your baby's growth and development. These dangerous consequences include inadequate brain growth, neurologic deficits, reading delays, bone loss, problems with coordination, developmental delays, difficulty with friendships and socializing, and many others. These serious and often permanent consequences may not be noticeable immediately, and, by the time they are evident, it can be too late to reverse the effects on your child's normal growth and development.

Caution: Sharing Breast Milk with Friends

If you're considering obtaining breast milk from a friend or asking a friend to breastfeed your baby, be sure to talk to your pediatric care provider about this first because breast milk is considered a living nutrient. A friend's breast milk may have the right nutrients for her baby, but not for yours. It can also contain dangerous bacteria and viruses that may pose a risk to your baby. Use trusted sources of information and be well informed before you make this choice that can have effects on your child's long-term health.

CHAPTER 14

Weaning Your Baby

Weaning is a personal decision influenced by many factors, some of which may be completely out of your control. Sometimes a mom is ready to stop and her baby isn't. Sometimes the baby decides that she wants to stop breastfeeding when she starts eating solids or her mom goes back to work. Others seem to want to continue breastfeeding until they go to pre-school, and others will wean themselves before their first birthday. There are as many different scenarios as there are babies and moms. If a baby weans and starts refusing to breastfeed before a mom is ready to stop, she may feel sad, depressed, frustrated, or angry.

It's normal to have mixed and conflicting feelings about weaning, especially if your experience with breastfeeding wasn't what you wanted or expected. It's important to let go of any guilt you might be feeling if you decide to wean, or if your milk supply is reduced and you have to wean. If you aren't able to provide breast milk for your baby, infant formula is the best and safest alternative.

Weaning is another topic that invites a lot of unsolicited advice from well-meaning people. You're the expert for your baby, which makes you the best person to decide when it's appropriate.

The following are some tips for how to wean your baby:

- First, consider how many times each day you breastfeed and look at the typical times.
- The last breastfeeding sessions to skip should be the very first and the very last of the day. Many moms find that they have weaned their baby completely except for a goodnight feeding before bedtime.
- Start by substituting a breastfeeding session with a bottle-feeding session in the midafternoon.
- Wait three days and then substitute a midmorning breastfeeding session with a bottle-feeding session.
- Every three days, substitute another breastfeeding session for a bottle-feeding session.
- By waiting three days between each eliminated breastfeeding session, you can avoid engorgement and painful breasts.
- For babies who aren't ready to give up breastfeeding, a mom will need help from her partner and family to provide the baby with a bottle, while she is in another room or out of the house.
- Some babies will tug at the breast and be very insistent on breastfeeding. As much as possible, if you're ready to wean, then hold them close, rock them, and offer a bottle,

a pacifier, or your clean finger as a substitute. They will eventually get used to your new routine. Remember, you're the mom and you're helping them grow and develop, even if they don't understand or accept these changes.

Enjoy Your Baby!

I hope that this booklet has been helpful as you feed your little one and she grows in her first year. This is a magical time for you, your baby, and your entire family. There are many paths to the same destination—a happy, healthy baby and a happy, healthy mom. If you need more tips and advice, see the listings in Useful Websites in the back of book. They have a lot more to offer.
Take care and enjoy your little one!

Checklist for When to Call Your Provider

- ❑ Your baby has less than five to eight wet diapers each day.
- ❑ Your baby has less than one stool each day.
- ❑ Your baby has a red rash on his or her bottom.
- ❑ You cannot wake your baby to breastfeed.
- ❑ Your baby cries at the breast and cannot latch on.
- ❑ Your baby breastfeeds for less than five minutes.
- ❑ Your baby breastfeeds for more than one hour.
- ❑ The mom's breasts are always engorged and the baby can't latch on.
- ❑ There is blood or pus coming out of one or both nipples.
- ❑ There is blood in your baby's diaper.

Useful Websites

Breastfeeding.com A great breastfeeding resource for all moms.

BreastfeedingInc.com Dr. Jack Newman's website with videos and helpful tips in many languages.

Ilca.org International Lactation Consultant Association, where you can find a certified lactation consultant.

KellyMom.com A resource with information and breastfeeding support forums.

Lalecheleague.org Breastfeeding information, support, and a way to find local support groups in your area.

NurseBarb.com Nurse Barb's website with helpful information on all aspects of women's health and parenting.

Postpartum.net Postpartum Support International, a resource for postpartum blues and depression.

Index

About the Author

Barb Dehn, R.N., M.S., N.P., is a women's health nurse practitioner in private practice and a much sought-after television commentator on health issues. She earned a master's degree from the University of California, San Francisco, and a bachelor of science degree from Boston College. Barb is certified as a menopause practitioner by the North American Menopause Society and is a Fellow in the American Association of Nurse Practitioners.

In addition to national appearances on CNN, NBC, and CBS, Nurse Barb, as she is known, took the extraordinary leap of bringing her blog, Nurse Barb's Daily Dose, to national television via ABC television. She is the award-winning author of a series of guides to women's health that are used by millions of women in the United States.

Barb lives in the San Francisco Bay area with her husband and son.

www.ingramcontent.com/pod-product-compliance
Lightning Source LLC
Jackson TN
JSHW071430200426
PP14546700006B/8

* 9 7 8 1 5 9 1 2 0 3 8 6 5 *

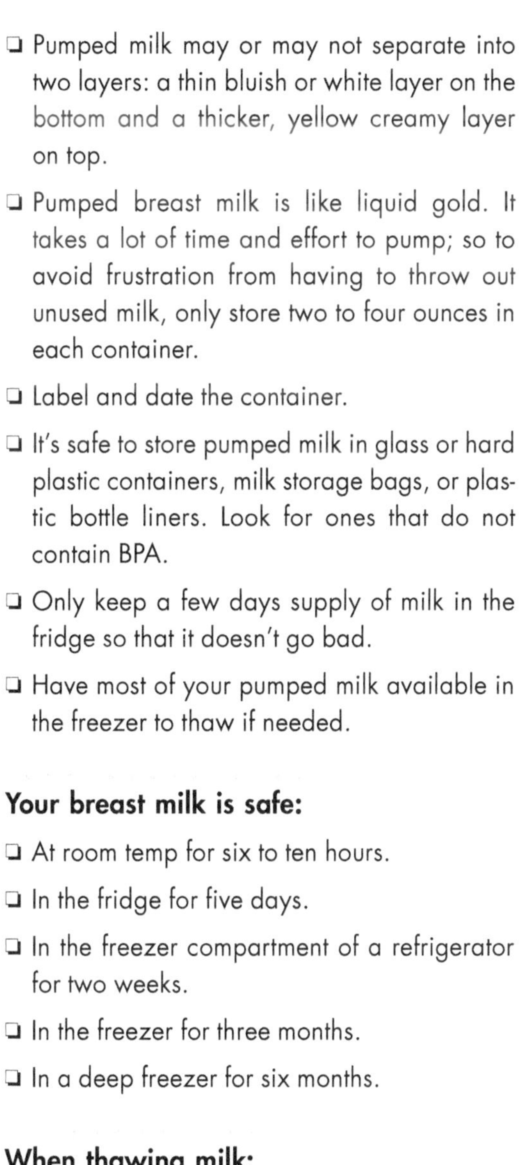

* 9 7 8 1 5 9 1 2 0 3 8 6 5 *